Trigger Point Therapy

Workbook for

Chest and Abdominal Pain

Valerie DeLaune, LAc

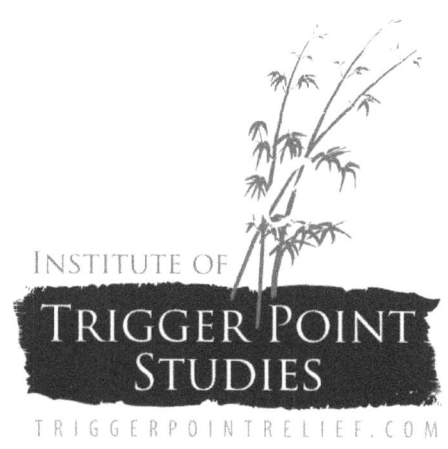

Copyright © 2024 by Valerie DeLaune. All rights reserved. No portion of this book, except for brief review, may be reproduced, stored in a retrieval system, or transmitted in any form or by any means – electronic, mechanical, photocopying, recording or otherwise – with the exception of downloading and purchase as an book and the device for which it was intended, without the written permission of the publisher. For information, contact the Institute of Trigger Point Studies at http://triggerpointrelief.com/.

ISBN 13: 978-0-9968553-8-9

Disclaimer:
The following information is intended for general information purposes only. Individuals should always see their health care provider before administering any suggestions made in this book. Any application of the material set forth in the following pages is at the reader's discretion and is his or her sole responsibility.

This book is intended as a quick-reference only for the major muscles that may harbor trigger points that refer pain to the chest and abdominal areas. It is not intended as a comprehensive therapy guide for other areas of the body. If you are unable to relieve all of your pain with the techniques found in this book, you may wish to consult one of the resources found at the end of this book in order to treat other pertinent muscles.

Table of Contents

Acknowledgements / About the Author 1

Chapter 1: Locating and Treating Trigger Points: General Guidelines 3

Chapter 2: Trigger Point Location Guide 10

Chapter 3: Paraspinals 13

Chapter 4: Quadratus Lumborum 24

Chapter 5: Pectoralis Major / Subclavius 31

Chapter 6: Pectoralis Minor 38

Chapter 7: Sternalis 41

Chapter 8: Sternocleidomastoid 44

Chapter 9: Scalenes 50

Chapter 10: Intercostals / Diaphragm 56

Chapter 11: Abdominals 62

Chapter 12: Adductor Muscles of the Hip 71

Chapter 13: Pelvic Floor 77

Appendix A: Perpetuating Factors 81

Other Books by the Author 101

Acknowledgements

This book would not have been possible without the lifeworks of Dr. Janet Travell and Dr. David G. Simons, who worked endlessly to research trigger points, document referral patterns and other symptoms, and bring all of that information to medical practitioners and the general public. Together Doctors Travell and Simons produced a comprehensive two-volume text on the causes and treatment of trigger points, written for physicians. This text is a condensation of those volumes, written for the general public, and for practitioners who don't need the in-depth knowledge to perform trigger point injections.

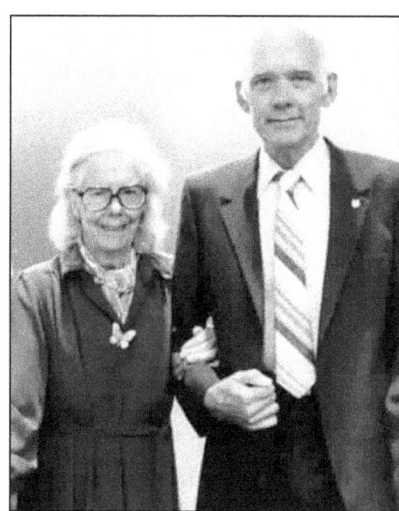

Dr. Janet Travell and Dr. David G. Simons

Dr. Travell pioneered and researched new pain treatments, including trigger point injections. In her private practice, she began treating Senator John F. Kennedy, who at the time was using crutches due to crippling back pain and was almost unable to walk down just a few stairs. It had become important for presidential candidates to appear physically fit, because of television. Being on crutches probably would have cost President Kennedy the election. Dr. Travell became the first female White House physician, and after President Kennedy died, she stayed on to treat President Johnson. She resigned a year and a half later to return to her passions: teaching, lecturing, and writing about chronic myofascial pain. She continued to work into her nineties and died at the age of ninety-five on August 1, 1997.

Dr. Simons met Dr. Travell when she lectured at the School of Aerospace Medicine at Brooks Air Force Base in Texas in the 1960s. He soon teamed up with Dr. Travell and began researching the international literature for any references to the treatment of pain. There were a few others out there who were also discovering trigger points but using different terminology. He studied and documented the physiology of trigger points in both laboratory and clinical settings and tried to find scientific explanations for trigger points. He continued to research the physiology of trigger points, update the trigger point volumes he coauthored with Dr. Travell, and review trigger point research articles until his death at the age of 88 on April 5, 2010.

I am also profoundly grateful to my neuromuscular therapy instructor, Jeanne Aland, who taught me basics about trigger points, and introduced me to the books written by Doctors Travell and Simons. I was told Jeanne passed on a few years ago.

All three are well-missed. Those familiar with trigger points are extremely grateful for their hard work and dedication. Their work lives on through the hundreds of thousands of patients who have gotten relief because of their research and willingness to train others.

Other Thanks

Many additional researchers have contributed to the study of trigger points, and many doctors and other practitioners have taken the time to learn about trigger points and give that information to their patients. I would like to acknowledge all of them for their role in alleviating pain by making this important information available. In particular I would like to thank Dr. Juhani Partanen, who kindly explained the "Muscle Spindle" hypothesis to me in lay terms, and also took the time to review the chapter "Trigger Points -- What Are They and What Causes Them?" to make sure I had translated scientific language correctly into easier-to-understand terms (this chapter is found in *Pain Relief with Trigger Point Self-Help*).

My Background

I attended massage school in 1989 and learned Swedish massage. I learned to give a very good general massage, but I didn't feel equipped to treat chronic pain. I was very intrigued by a description of a continuing education certificate course; it was called *neuromuscular therapy*, which combines *myofascial release* (a type of deep tissue massage) with treating trigger points. I attended the class in 1991, taught by Jeanne Aland at Heartwood Institute, and it completely changed my approach to treating patients. Once I learned about referral patterns, I was able to consistently resolve chronic pain problems.

Over my years of treating thousands of patients, I have added my own observations to those of Doctors Travell and Simons, and developed a variety of self-help techniques, which are included in my books.

In 1999, I received my master's degree in acupuncture. Since then I've been writing trigger point books and articles, teaching trigger point continuing education classes to health care providers, and specializing in treating pain syndromes by combining dry-needling of trigger points with Traditional Chinese Medicine diagnosis and treatment.

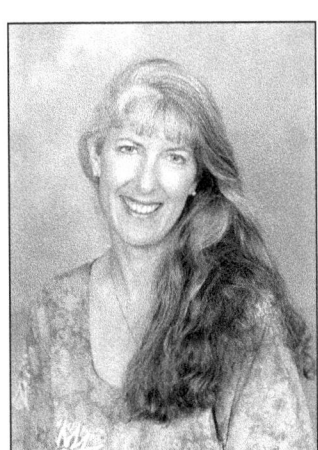
Valerie DeLaune, LAc

Chapter 1: Locating and Treating Trigger Points: General Guidelines

***If you are experiencing sudden chest or abdominal pain,
go to the emergency room!***

While trigger points can cause a great deal of pain that feels like it is in an organ, it is imperative to get serious conditions ruled out first and then work on trigger points later. You should see a medical provider *immediately* to rule out serious conditions if you have pain with any of the following symptoms:

- Your pain had a sudden onset, is severe, or starts with a traumatic injury, particularly if it is in your chest or abdomen, or radiating from the chest down your arms.

- You develop poor circulation, painful varicose veins, and very cold legs, feet, arms, or hands.

- Your pain is accompanied by a fever, redness, heat, severe swelling, or odd sensations.

- Your pain lasts for more than two weeks, unless you have already ruled out more serious conditions.

- The intensity of pain increases over time, or the symptoms are different; changes can be an indication of a different, more serious cause.

- You develop rashes or ulcers that don't heal.

Referred symptoms due to trigger points can mimic other, more serious conditions, or can occur concurrently with them. It may take some investigation to determine the ultimate cause of the problem. Most muscle chapters in this book contain a section labeled "Differential Diagnosis." Unless you are a health care provider, it's likely you won't understand most of what it says. Don't be too concerned about this; the section has been included so that you can take it to a health care provider and be evaluated for those conditions, though you still ought to read it.

Hopefully your health care provider will rule out any serious conditions. If you are diagnosed with pain from structural damage or chronic conditions, chances are you can relieve much or all of your pain with a combination of self-treatment of trigger points and addressing and eliminating the perpetuating factors. Regardless of the diagnosis you receive from a health care provider, my general treatment principle is the same: identify and eliminate all the underlying perpetuating causes to the extent possible *after any critical danger has passed*, and treat the trigger points.

Copyright © 2024 Valerie DeLaune, LAc

Where to Start?

Chapter 2 contains the *Trigger Point Location Guide;* this will help you figure out which muscles in this book may harbor trigger points that might be causing your symptoms. Locate your pain or other symptoms for each area, and then refer to the chapters listed.

Each muscle chapter has drawings that show the most common pain referral areas for each trigger point. The more solid black or white area indicates the primary area of referral, which is almost always present, and the lighter stippled area shows the most likely secondary areas of referral, which may or may not be present. Keep in mind that the referral patterns only show the most *common* referral patterns; your referral pattern may be somewhat different or even completely different. You may also have overlapping referral patterns from trigger points in multiple muscles. These areas may be more extensive than the patterns common for individual muscles, and pain may be more intense. For this reason, over time, be sure to search for trigger points in all the muscles that refer pain to that area.

Each muscle chapter contains an anatomical drawing of the muscle or muscles covered in that chapter, with "X"'s showing some of the most common locations of trigger points. *There may be additional trigger points or they may be in different places, so search the entire muscle.* Keep in mind that for some muscles, the "X" may just be an *example* of a trigger point location and its associated referral pattern, but they may occur at any level; for example, trigger points in the *paraspinal* muscles.

Each muscle chapter also includes lists of common symptoms and factors that may cause or perpetuate trigger points. Again, these are only the most common; you may experience different symptoms, and your causes and perpetuating factors may be different. If you think you might have trigger points in a certain muscle but don't see any perpetuating factors that apply to you, try to imagine whether anything in your life is similar to something on the list that could be causing the same type of stress on the muscle.

Once you've determined which two muscles most closely fit your pain referral pattern and symptoms, start doing the self-help pressure and stretching, and eliminate the applicable perpetuating factors. Over the next several weeks, search for trigger points in additional muscles, and add those into your treatment regime as needed. As you start to feel better, you'll develop a clearer picture of which trigger points are causing your pain, and which perpetuating factors are reactivating your trigger points.

Other Things to Consider...

When you apply pressure to the trigger point, you can often reproduce the referred pain or other symptoms, but being unable to reproduce the referred pain or other symptoms by applying pressure does *not* rule out involvement of that specific trigger point. Try treating the trigger points that could be causing the problem anyway, and if you improve, even temporarily, assume that one of the trigger points you worked on is indeed at least part of the problem. For this reason, don't work on all the possible trigger points in one session, since you won't know which trigger point treated actually gave you relief.

Be aware that a *primary*, or *key*, trigger point can cause a *satellite* trigger point to develop in a different muscle. The satellite trigger point may have formed for one of these reasons: it lies within the referral zone of the primary trigger point, or it's in a muscle that is either substituting for, or is countering tension for the muscle that contains the primary trigger point. When doing self-treatments, be aware that if some of your trigger points are satellite trigger points, you won't get lasting relief until the primary trigger points have been treated. This is why it is important to work in the direction of referral (see "Do's" below).

You also need to be aware that central sensitization (explained in *Pain Relief with Trigger Point Self-Help*) can cause the referral pattern to deviate from the most common pattern found in each muscle chapter. It may also cause trigger points in several muscles within a region to refer pain to the same area, making it more difficult to determine trigger point locations. This means you can't absolutely rule out the role of a potential trigger point based *only* on consideration of common referral patterns, since other factors may cause you to have an *uncommon* referral pattern. The more intense the earlier pain, the more intense the emotions associated with it, and the longer pain has lasted, the more likely central sensitization will cause deviation from the most common referral patterns.

A small percentage of people will get worse before they get better, mostly in complex cases. Or the pain may move around, or you may have the perception that the pain moved around only because the most painful areas have improved and now you are noticing the next most painful area more. I've only had a few cases where I wasn't able to help patients, because they were so frustrated after receiving little or no help from professional after professional that they only allowed me to treat them a few times before giving up, *even if they had improved*. If you get a little worse before you get better, you may be inclined to give up in the initial stages of treatment. I encourage you to give any treatment you try some amount of time before you decide it isn't working, even if your condition initially gets worse.

General Guidelines for Applying Self-Pressure

DON'Ts:

- **Do not apply pressure over varicose veins, open wounds, infections, herniated/bulging disks, areas of phlebitis/thrombophlebitis, or where clots are present or could be present. If you are pregnant, do not apply pressure on your legs.**

- **Most importantly: *Don't overdo the self-help techniques!*** Many people think that if some feels great, more will be even better, but you can actually make yourself worse by not following the guidelines. Expect gradual improvement, though you may improve most quickly during the initial weeks of therapy.

DO's:

- **Use a tennis ball, racquetball, golf ball, dog play ball, or baseball, or use your elbow or hand if instructed for particular muscles.** For balls, use the weight of your body to give you the pressure; don't press your back or limb onto the balls. The muscle you are working on should be as passive as possible. Use one ball at a time on your back, not one on each side.

- **Apply pressure for a minimum of eight seconds, and a maximum of one minute;** less than eight seconds may activate trigger points, and more than a minute will cut off the circulation for too long and make it worse. Time yourself first to be sure you are actually counting seconds at the correct speed.

- **It should be somewhat uncomfortable, or "hurt good," but it should not be so painful that you are either tensing up or holding your breath. If it is too painful, use a smaller or softer ball, or move to a softer surface (like a bed, or pad your surface with a pillow or blanket).** If it does *not* hurt at all, keep looking for tender spots, or try moving to a harder surface. If it's too tender to lie on, try putting a ball in a long sock and leaning against the wall. I only recommend using the wall if you cannot lie on the ball, since you are then using the very muscles you are trying to work on. You may need to use a combination of surfaces depending on the tenderness of different areas. Over time, as sensitivity decreases, you may need to change ball dimensions and/or hardness, or move to a harder surface.

- **Search the *entire* muscle for tender points, particularly the points of maximum tenderness.** Use the pictures to make sure you are getting the entire muscle and not just the worst spot. Many times a tendon attachment will hurt because the tight muscle is pulling on it, but if you don't treat the bulk of the muscle, it will keep pulling on the attachment.

- **Be sure to work on both sides of the body to keep the muscles balanced, but spend more time on the areas that need it more.** Except for very new one-sided injuries, the same muscle on the opposite side will almost always be tender with pressure, even if it has not yet started causing symptoms. If you loosen one side but not the other, it can lead to additional problems. Sometimes problems with the muscles on the opposite side are actually causing the symptoms, so it is always worth working on both sides.

- **Work in the direction of referral.** For example, if your abdominal muscles hurt and the pain is being referred from trigger points in the paraspinal muscles in the back, work on the back first, then your abdominal area.

- If you have limited time, **do one area thoroughly rather than rushing through many areas**. You are more likely to aggravate trigger points rather than inactivate them if you rush.

- **Do stretches *after* the trigger point work.** If you only have time to do one thing, do the ball/pressure work and skip the stretches.

- **Most people should work on their muscles one time per day initially**. If you have an appointment with your therapist, do not do your self-help the same day. If you are sore from your therapy appointment or your self-help, skip a day. If you are sore for more than one day or your symptoms get worse, it is likely that either the pressure was too hard or you held points for too long. Review these guidelines if that is the case. Tell your therapist if you are sore from their work. This is *not* a case of where if some is great, more is better.

    Pick a time when you will remember to do your self-help, i.e., when you wake up, when you watch television, or when you go to bed, and keep your balls by the bed (*but do not fall asleep on a ball!*).

    After a few weeks, you may wish to increase your self-help to twice per day, as long as you are not getting sore. If a particular activity bothers you, you may wish to do the self-help before and after the activity. If you start getting sore or your symptoms get worse, decrease your self-help frequency.

    Treat your trigger points for as long as they are sensitive, even if active symptoms have disappeared. If trigger points are still tender, they are *latent*, and could easily be reactivated. Most likely you will start forgetting as symptoms disappear; however, the most important thing you will have learned is what to do if your symptoms return.

- **If you have questions or your symptoms get worse, or you are sore for more than one day, stop the self-help until you have had a chance to consult with your therapist**. They should be able to help you figure out any problems.

- **Take your balls on trips with you**, since travel frequently aggravates trigger points. You may even wish to keep some balls at work.

General Guidelines for Stretches and Conditioning

It is very important to distinguish the difference between *stretching* and *conditioning* exercises. *Stretching* means you gently lengthen the muscle fibers. *Conditioning* means you are trying to strengthen the muscle. Doctors Travell and Simons found that *active* trigger points benefited from stretching, but were usually aggravated by conditioning exercises. Once trigger points have been *inactivated*, conditioning is beneficial. Make sure your physical therapist or physiotherapist is familiar with trigger points, and begins your therapy with stretching exercises.

Usually two weeks of trigger point self-help treatment will be sufficient before adding in conditioning exercises, but if your trigger points are still very irritable, you will need to wait until your symptoms improve. Meanwhile, learn the stretches in this book. If you are not sure whether an assigned activity is a stretch or conditioning, ask your practitioner. I will not cover guidelines for conditioning exercises in depth here, since your physical therapist or physiotherapist will prescribe them.

DON'Ts:

- **Don't bounce on stretches, and avoid stretching when your muscles are tired or cold.**

- **Don't do a conditioning exercise just because it worked for someone else.** Doctors Travell and Simons said "Exercise should be regarded as a prescription, much as one prescribes medication. Like a drug, there is a right kind, dose, and timing of exercise." Often a friend will recommend an exercise that worked for them, but you are a different person with a different set of symptoms, and you should no more do their assigned exercises than you would take their prescribed medications. Be sure to tell your therapist all of the activities and exercises/stretches you are doing, because one of these can be contributing to your trigger point activation.

- **Don't keep doing an exercise or stretch that is aggravating your symptoms.** Check with your therapist to determine why it is bothering you and to find out how to proceed.

DO's:

- **Stretch slowly, and only to the point of just getting a gentle stretch; *don't force it*.** If you stretch the muscles too hard or too fast, you can aggravate trigger points.

- **Hold your stretch for 30 to 60 seconds.** There will be little benefit after 30 seconds, but it will not hurt you to stretch for longer either. You may repeat the stretch after releasing and breathing.

- **For any type of repetitive exercise, breathe and rest between each cycle of the exercise.**

- **If you are sore for more than one day** from exercises or stretches, reduce the number of repetitions and try again after the soreness has disappeared. If you are still sore for two days after the exercise or stretch, it needs to be changed.

General Guidelines for Muscle Care

These are some general suggestions for taking care of your muscles; each muscle chapter will have specific suggestions.

DON'Ts:

- Never put the maximum load on a muscle -- it is too easy to strain it.

- Don't lift something too heavy -- ask for help.

- Don't keep muscles in positions of sustained contractions, where you are holding them tense or in sustained use. In order to increase blood flow and bring oxygen and nutrients to the muscles, they need to alternately constrict and relax.

- Don't sit for too long in one position.

- Don't expose your muscles to cold drafts.

DO's:

- After treatments, gently use the muscle in a normal way that uses its full range-of-motion, but avoid strenuous activities immediately afterward or until the trigger points aren't so easily aggravated, whichever is longer.

- Vary your activities so you are not doing any one thing for too long. Rest and take breaks frequently from any given activity.

- Lift with your knees bent and your back straight, with the object close to your chest.

- Notice where you hold tension and practice relaxing those areas.

- Swimming is generally a good exercise, and bicycling is easier on the body than running, but in both cases, take care to avoid straining the trapezius and neck muscles. A recumbent, stationary, or other bike that allows you to sit more upright is preferable.

- When starting an exercise program, *underestimate* what you will be able to do. Gradually add increments in duration, rate, and effort, and in amounts that will not cause you to be sore or activate trigger points.

- Warm-up adequately for sports activities.

- If you are working with a practitioner, they should be able to help you prioritize what needs to be done in order of most importance. If your practitioner is giving you too many things to do at once, be sure to tell them that you are overwhelmed and need to set priorities. Giving a patient too many assignments is all too easy for a practitioner to do, especially when they are first out of school and brimming with many useful ideas and suggestions.

Copyright © 2024 Valerie DeLaune, LAc

Be sure to return to this chapter often to review the guidelines to ensure you are treating the muscles properly, particularly if something is not working for you, or trigger points are getting aggravated instead of inactivated. Chances are you have forgotten to follow these guidelines.

Be sure to set realistic goals. Focus on a few muscles at a time unless there is a reason that you need to work on several together. Setting unrealistic goals can discourage you, and cause you to give up. It's better to pick just a few things and do them well rather than rush through too many self-help techniques or suggestions and do them poorly. You probably won't be able to apply pressure on five different muscles and stretch them, get orthotics and replace bad shoes, change your diet, and start walking every day all in the first week. Pace yourself so that this is an enjoyable process, and work on the perpetuating factors over time.

Chapter 2: Trigger Point Location Guide

To figure out which muscles to work on first, look at the trigger point location guides and refer to the chapters listed for each. Examine the photos of referral patterns in each chapter and try to find those that most closely match your pain pattern, and read the list of symptoms for each muscle. Refer to chapter 1 for additional instructions on locating and treating trigger points, and general guidelines for applying pressure, stretching, and general muscle care.

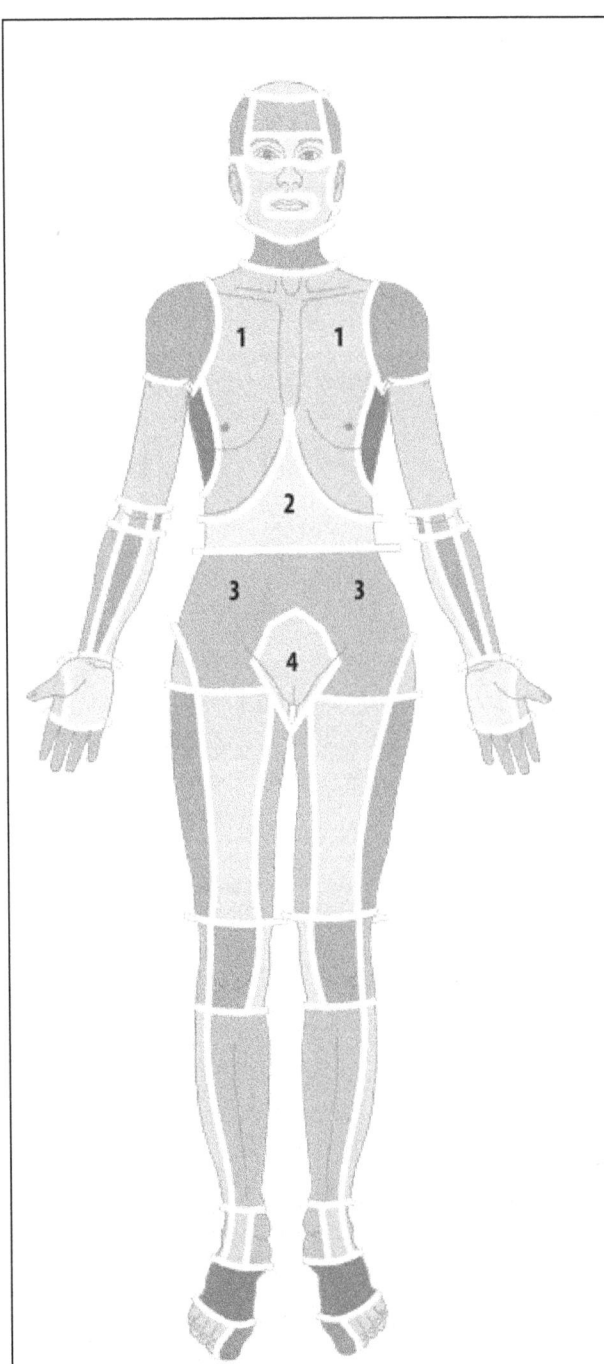

1. Pectoralis major / Subclavius (5)
   Pectoralis minor (6)
   Scalene (9)
   Sternocleidomastoid (8)
   Sternalis (7)
   Intercostals / Diaphragm (10)
   Iliocostalis cervicis (3)
   External abdominal oblique (11)

2. Abdominal (11)
   Paraspinals (3)
   Quadratus lumborum (4)

3. Abdominal (11)
   Paraspinals (3)
   Quadratus lumborum (4)

4. Pelvic floor (13)
   Adductor magnus (12)
   Abdominal (11)

Muscle chapters for all of the remaining areas of the body can be found in *Pain Relief with Trigger Point Self-Help*. Please see the end of this book for more information.

Blank Body Chart

You may wish to make copies of the following blank body chart and draw your symptom pattern on one of them with a colored marker. Then you can compare your pattern with the pain referral pictures in chapters 3 through 13. Out to the side of each painful area, note your pain intensity on a scale of 1 to 10 and the percent of time you feel pain in that area—for example, 6.5/80%.

I recommend that you fill out a body chart at least a couple of times per week. Date them so that you'll be able to keep them in order. This chronological record will come in handy in several ways. It will:

- make it easier for you to discern which patterns fit your pain referral most closely;
- help you recognize the factors that cause and perpetuate your symptoms by matching fluctuations in the level and frequency of your symptoms;
- allow you to track your progress (or lack thereof) and provide a historical record of any injuries.

As your condition improves, you may forget how intense your symptoms were originally, and you may think you're not getting any better. You'll be able to see that you are improving, even if you have an occasional setback. One thing to note, however, is that not everyone can accurately draw their pain location, due in part to lack of familiarity with anatomy, so take that possibility into consideration and check muscles with adjacent referral patterns just in case your drawing is inaccurate.

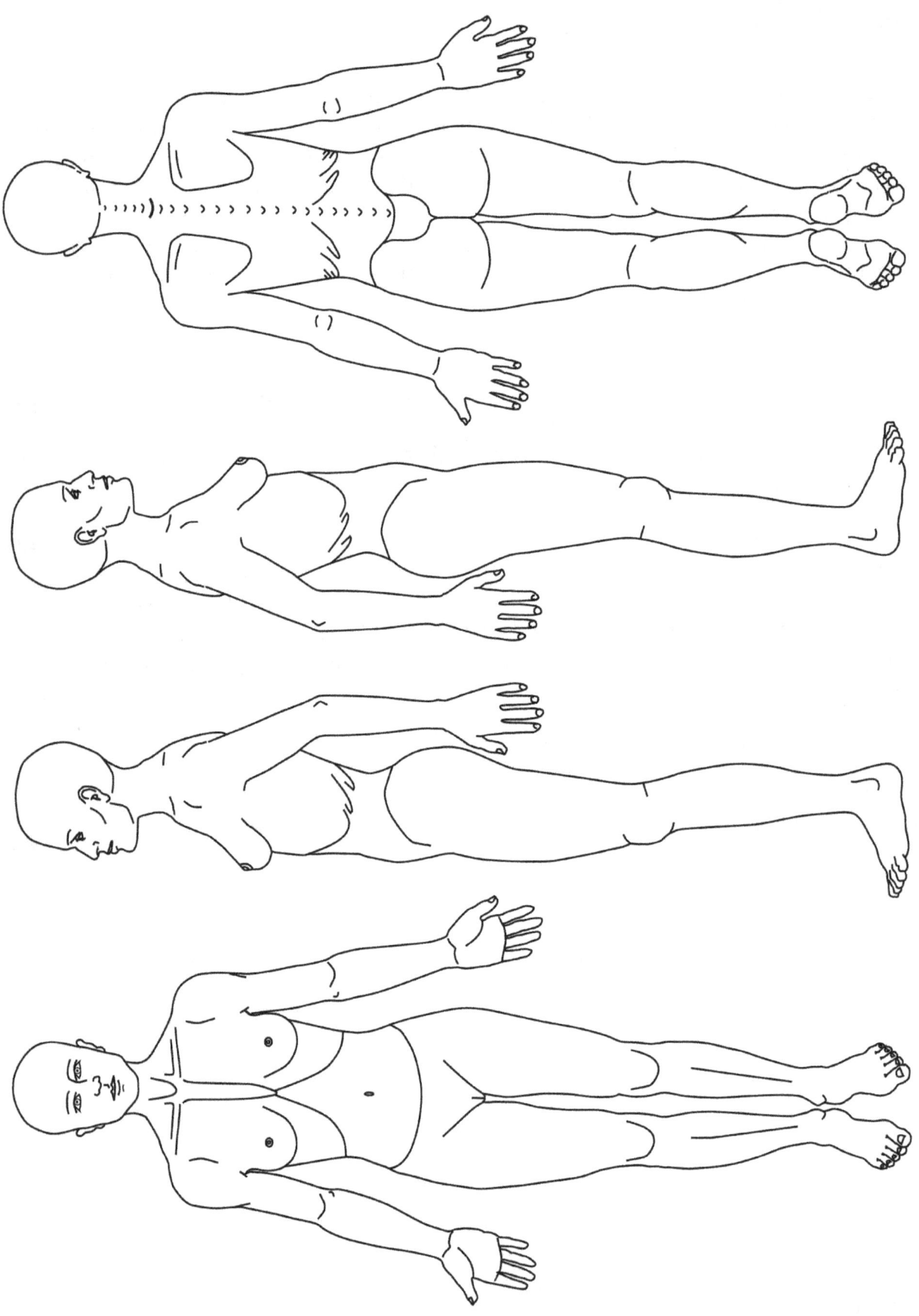

Chapter 3: Paraspinals
(Iliocostalis Lumborum, Cervicis, & Thoracis,
Longissimus Thoracis, Multifidi)

Part of this muscle group runs the entire length of the spine, and some of the muscles run most of the length of the spine. Yet others (the *multifidi*) are small muscles that attach one vertebra to the next. These are the muscles that allow you to bend and twist.

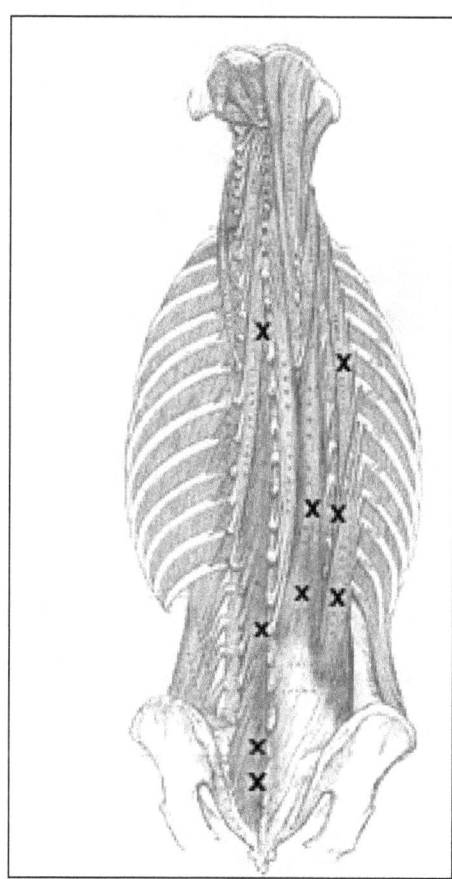
Back view of trunk

Common Symptoms

- See the pictures for all the pain referral patterns. These pictures show common trigger points, **but trigger points can develop <u>at any level</u> and cause similar referral patterns <u>at any level</u>**. Please note that in many cases pain can refer to the front side of the body, causing you to think you are having organ problems, particularly in the area of the heart. Trigger points in these muscles are an often overlooked cause of buttocks pain.
- deep, aching pain that feels like it is in the spine
- pain may increase with coughing or straining to have a bowel movement
- restricted range-of-motion or restricted rotation of the trunk, possibly severe
- possibly difficulty climbing stairs or getting out of a chair
- possibly nausea, belching, and gastrointestinal pain and cramping

- entrapment of spinal nerves cause increased or decreased sensitivity and/or uncomfortable sensations on the skin of the back
- stiffness in the spine, mostly from the *longissimus thoracis*

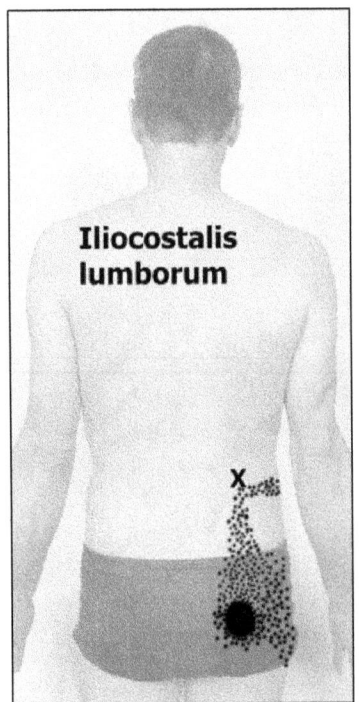
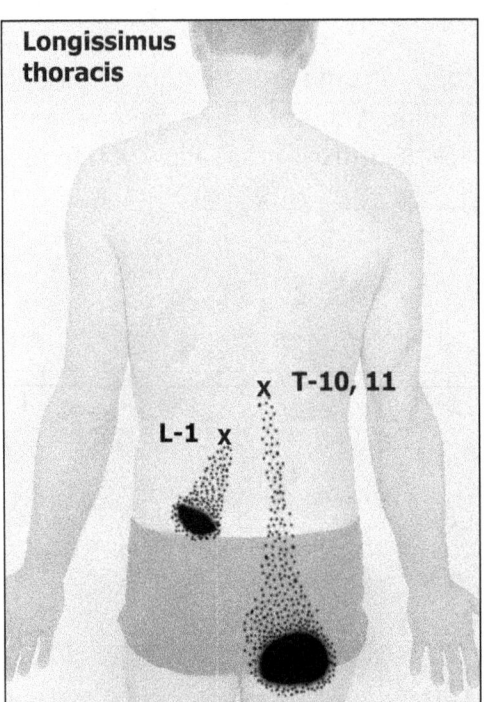

Sample referral patterns, but all of these can occur at any level of the back.

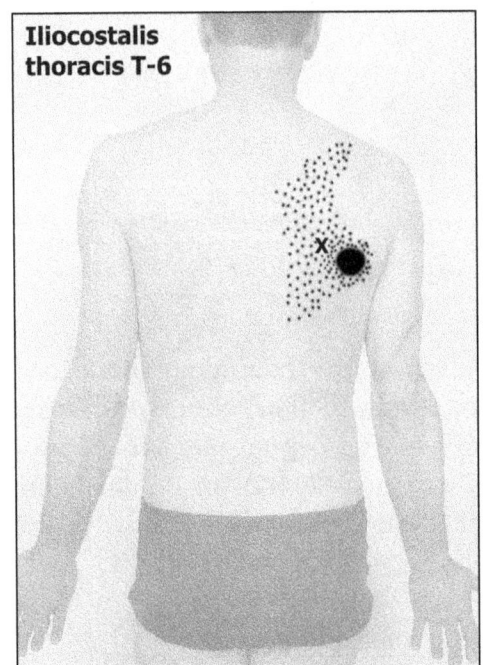

Back referral pattern

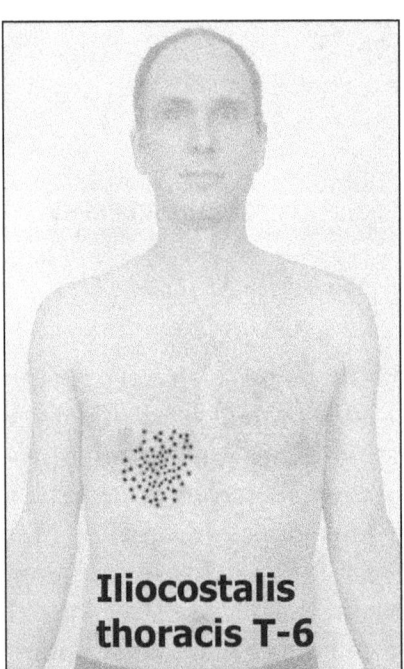

Front referral pattern

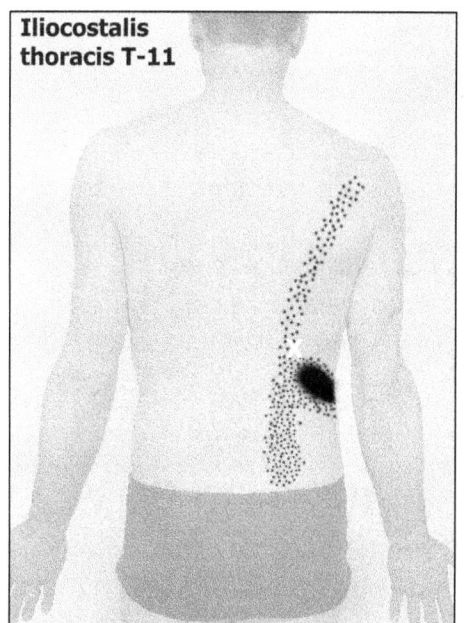
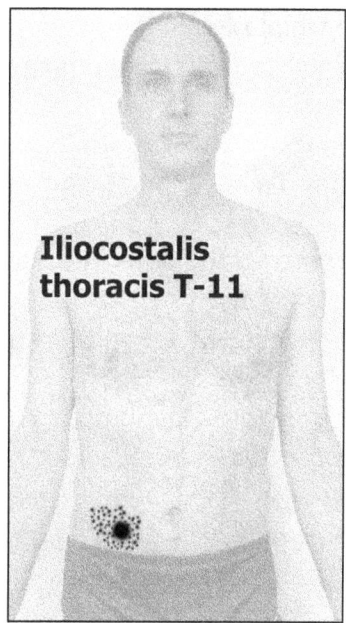

Sample referral patterns, but all of these can occur at any level of the back.

Back referral pattern   Front referral pattern

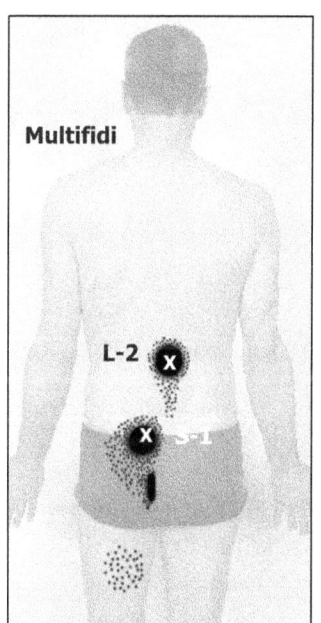
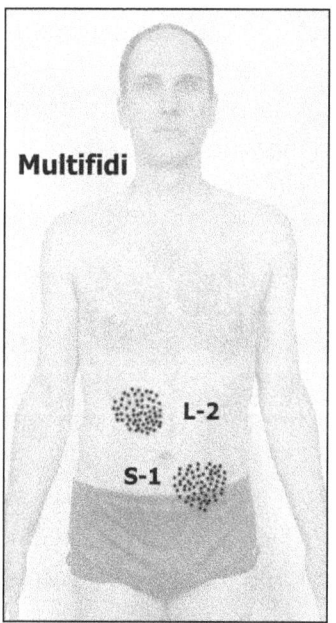
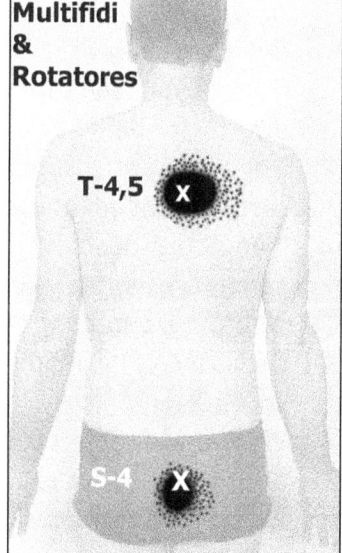

Back referral pattern   Front referral pattern

Causes and Perpetuation of Trigger Points

- a sudden overload, often when bending, lifting, and twisting at the same time (people frequently tell me they were moving boxes)
- catching yourself from falling, such as when slipping on ice
- sitting for long periods without moving, in as little as hour or less for some people
- sitting on a wallet in your back pocket
- bending over while gardening
- injury is more likely when the muscles are chilled or fatigued

- car accidents, especially a whiplash injury
- mattresses that are too old or too soft, or sleeping next to someone who is heavier and trying to avoid rolling into them
- a tight belt or bra strap
- trigger points in the *latissimus dorsi* (a muscle covering the back and sides of the trunk)
- head-forward posture
- one leg anatomically shorter than the other (this does *not* refer to the "short leg" terminology chiropractors often use to describe the effect of vertebrae being out-of-alignment), or an unequal hemipelvis size (either the right or left half of the pelvis)

This is a list of perpetuating factors specific only to trigger points in these muscles. For a full list of perpetuating factors that can cause and perpetuate trigger points anywhere in the body and which also apply to these muscles, please see "Appendix A" (found at the end of this book), since some may need to be addressed for lasting pain relief.

Helpful Hints

- Don't keep a wallet in a back pocket, since it will tilt your pelvis and spine when sitting.
- Modify or replace your mis-fitting furniture. Your knees should fit under your desk, and the chair needs to be close enough that you can lean against your backrest. Your elbows should rest on either your work surface or armrests at the same height. Your elbows and forearms should rest evenly on the armrests. Your computer screen should be directly in front of you, and the copy attached to the side of the screen, so that you may look directly forward as much as possible. Take frequent breaks.
- Get a headset or speaker for your phone, or hold the phone with one hand. Shoulder rests are not adequate.
- If you must bend over plans or reading materials (such as a draftsman, engineer, or architect), a tilted work surface will alleviate the mechanical stress to a point, but be sure to take frequent breaks.
- Lift properly by bending your knees rather than your back, and hold objects close to your body.
- Wear bras that fit properly. If you see elastic marks on your skin after you take your bra off, the straps are too tight. Jogging bras work great for medium or small-breasted women. Have the salesperson help you find a bra that fits properly -- many of them really know their products.
- If you are gardening, straighten up frequently, and stand and stretch periodically.
- Be sure to slide into the center of your car seat. Some bucket seats curve up on each side, and if you are not in the center, your pelvis is tilted.
- Buy a firm mattress, and replace it every five to seven years. You can put plywood between the box springs and mattress to make it firmer.
- If you have difficulty getting up, roll over onto your hands and knees and crawl to where you can grab onto something and pull yourself up.
- When standing up from a chair, slide your butt to the front of the chair, turn your entire body a little sideways, put one foot under the front edge of the chair, then stand with

your torso erect so that your thighs take the load. You can use your hands to assist you if necessary. Sit down in the opposite sequence.
- When climbing stairs or a ladder, rotate your entire body 45-degrees and keep your back straight.
- Restoration of proper posture, especially head positioning, is critical to treating trigger points since head-forward posture can both cause and perpetuate trigger points. Head-forward posture can be aggravated while sitting in a car, at a desk, in front of a computer, or while eating dinner or watching TV. Using a good lumbar support everywhere you sit will help correct poor sitting posture. See the exercise below in the "Self-Help Techniques" section for postural re-training.

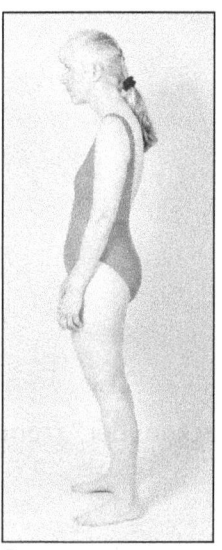
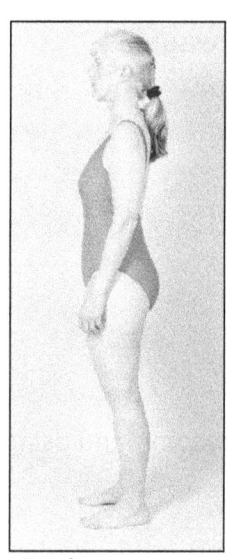

Poor posture   **Good Posture**

- If you have a body asymmetry or an anatomically shorter leg, see a specialist to get compensating lifts or pads.

Self-Help Techniques

Applying Pressure

Paraspinal Pressure: The shading on the picture marks the area you will want to work on.

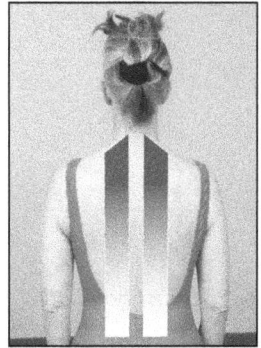

Lie face-up on a firm bed or the floor, with your knees bent. Using a tennis ball or racquet ball, start at the shoulder, about one inch out to the side of the spine, and hold pressure for eight seconds to one minute per spot. Shift a small amount to the next spot further down the back by using your legs to move your body over the ball, and continue to hold pressure on each spot. Continue working down all the way to the top of the pelvis in order to treat both the *trapezius* and the *paraspinal* muscles. You may want to repeat this on a second line further out from the spine, especially if you have a wide back or if you have tender points further out. *Do not do this directly on the spine!* I recommend using one ball at a time, rather than using a ball on each side at the same time. By performing this technique lying down, as opposed to standing and leaning into the wall, you keep the muscles as passive as possible, so that you are not using them to hold you upright while you are applying pressure.

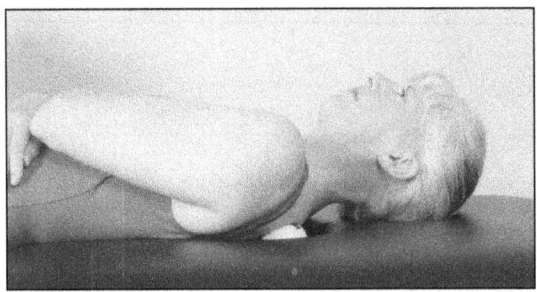

If you are at work and unable to lie on the floor, I recommend using a Backnobber® from Pressure Positive Company (see below).

Longissimus thoracis pressure: To work on the *longissimus thoracis*, which is very close to the spine, you will need to lie on a hard floor and use a golf ball. Place the golf ball *in between* your spine and the muscle (not *on* the spine—see photo), and then move your body just a little *away* from the side you are working on. This presses on the muscles at a 45° angle, the only really effective way to get this muscle. Do this from the bottom of the neck, down to the top of the pelvis. As a trigger point therapist, I perform this treatment by standing on the opposite side and leaning across, pressing the muscle out at a 45° angle.

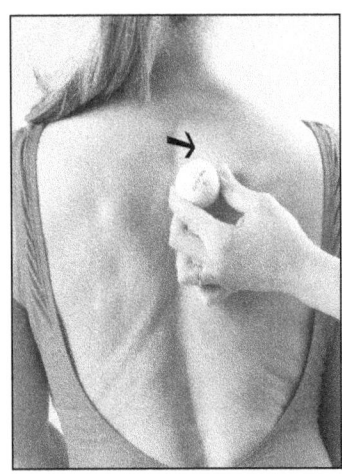

Demonstrating location of muscle and direction to press out against golf ball

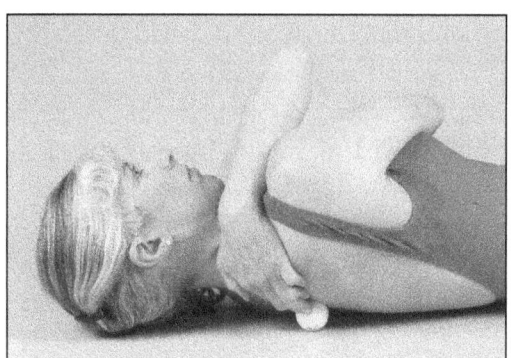 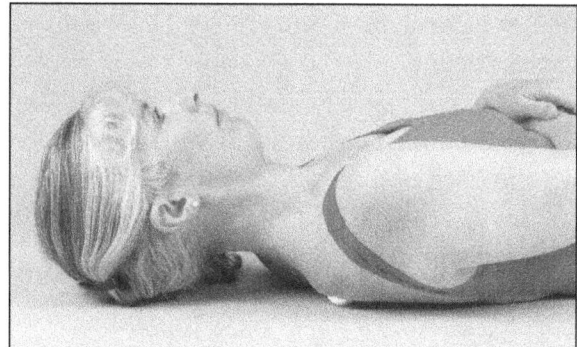

Lay on a golf ball to perform this self-help technique

Multifidi pressure: To treat the *multifidi* (the little muscles that attach one vertebra to the next), you will need the assistance of another person, as even a golf ball is too large. They will need a tool, such as a rubber-tipped wooden dowel (available at a massage supply store), or an eraser that is rounded off. Working next to the spinous process (the pointy part of the vertebra), massage in the groove next to it. Your assistant may be able to use their thumb, but a gadget works better and is easier on the person administering the treatment.

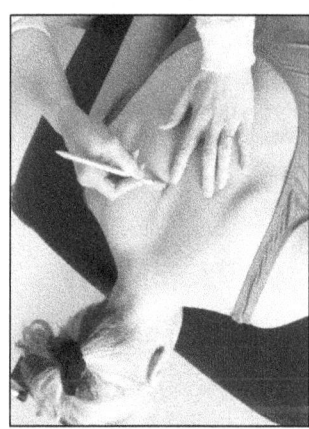

Backnobber®: If you are at work and unable to lie on the floor, I recommend using a Backnobber® from Pressure Positive Company to apply pressure to the *paraspinal* muscles. Note how both hands are pulling the Backnobber® away from the body in the direction the arrows are pointing, rather than pressing it into the front of the trunk to lever pressure onto the back.

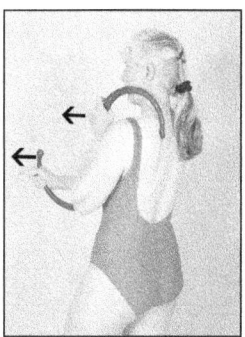

Copyright © 2024 Valerie DeLaune, LAc

Posterior Neck Pressure: I find it is best to treat the *paraspinal* muscles first and the *posterior neck* muscles second.

The shading in the picture marks the area to work on. You may work along the base of the skull and down the back of the neck. Try to get all the way to the base of the neck where it intersects the top of the shoulder, in order to work on the entire *splenius cervicis* and *iliocostalis cervicis* muscles.

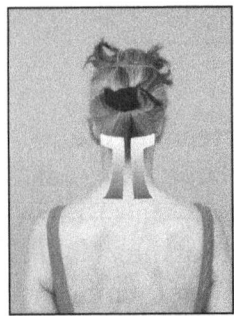

To treat the back of your neck, use a golf ball and lie face-up with your hands behind your neck. One palm should be squarely over the other palm, with the golf ball in the center of your top palm, and *not* where the fingers join the palm.

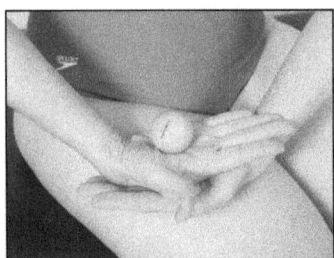

Keep your head relaxed throughout the self-treatment. To apply pressure, rotate your head toward the ball. Be sure to work on the muscles to the *side* of the spine—don't put the ball directly *on* the spine. To move the ball, roll your head away from the side you are working on, move the ball a small amount, and then rotate your head back toward the side you are working on. If you want more pressure, rotate your head toward the side you are working on even more; rotate your head less if you want less pressure. *Do not raise your head to move the ball.* This will cause additional stress on the muscles, so be sure to move the ball by *rotating* your head away from it.

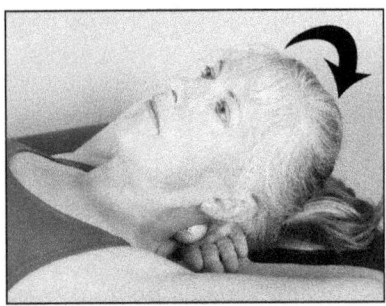

Copyright © 2024 Valerie DeLaune, LAc

Stretches

In-Bathtub Stretch: With your head hanging forward, lean forward and reach your hands down toward your toes, until you are feeling a gentle stretch. Relax and then repeat, moving your hands further down each time, but only as far down as you can feel a gentle stretch. Do this in a hot bath if you can. [**Note**: If you have trigger points in the *iliopsoas* muscle, even if they are latent, this stretch can cause a reactive cramp. You may need to work on and stretch the *iliopsoas* first, but since trigger points in the *iliopsoas* muscles don't directly cause chest or abdominal pain, they are not addressed in this book. Go to the end of this book for other books by the author that provide self-treatment techniques of muscles not covered in this book.]

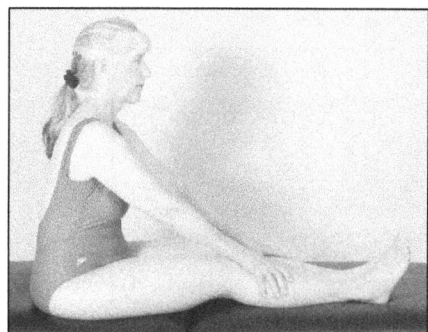
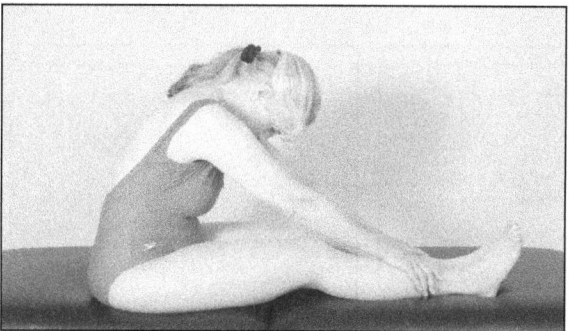
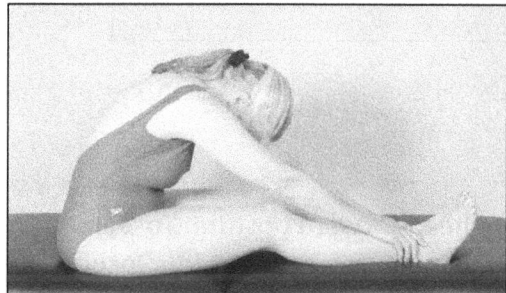
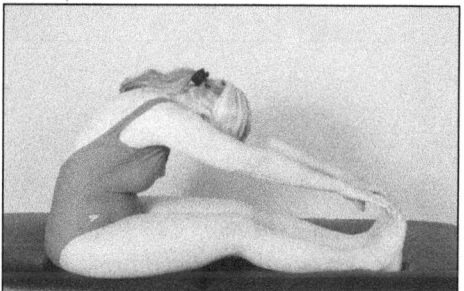

Low Back Stretching Exercise: Lying on your back, with your hands clasped *behind* one knee, gently bring that knee toward your chest until you are just feeling the stretch. Repeat with the opposite knee, and then both legs at the same time.

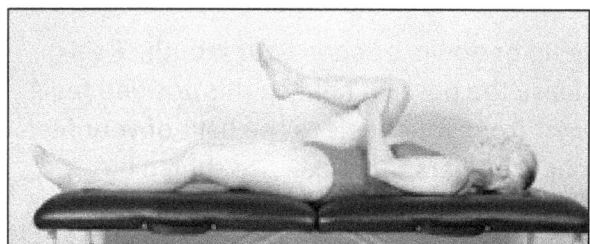
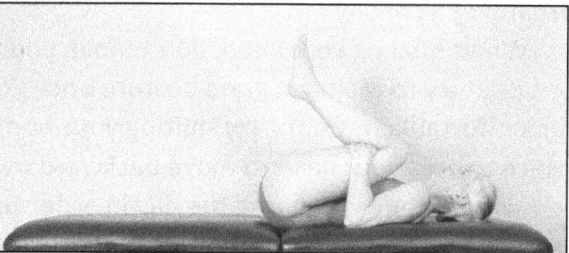

Copyright © 2024 Valerie DeLaune, LAc

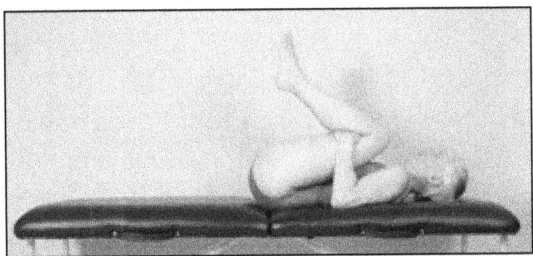

Posterior Neck Stretch: You may do this stretch under a hot shower and, if possible, seated on a stool. Lock your fingers behind your head and pull your head gently forward. Turn your head to one side at a 45° angle and gently pull your head in that direction. Place one hand on the top of your head and gently pull your head down to that side. Repeat on the opposite side.

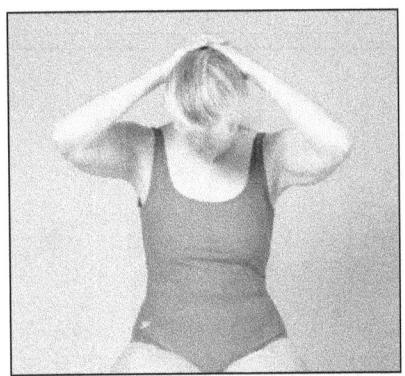 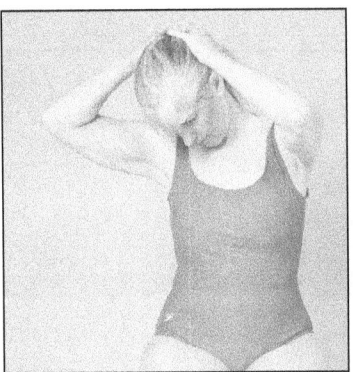 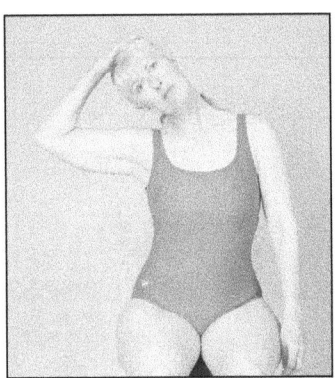

Exercises

Postural Re-training: Postural exercises can help eliminate head-forward posture. To learn proper posture and correct a head-forward position, stand with your feet about four inches apart, with your arms at your sides and thumbs pointing forward. Tighten your buttocks to stabilize your lower back, then, while inhaling, rotate your arms and shoulders out and back by rotating your thumbs backward, and squeeze the shoulder blades together in the back. Keep holding this position while dropping your shoulders down and exhaling. Move your head back to bring your ears in line with your shoulders and hold this position for about six seconds while breathing normally.

When moving your head, don't move your nose up or down, or open your mouth. Relax, but then try to maintain good posture once you release the pose. If holding this position feels uncomfortable or "stiff," try shifting your body weight from your heels to the balls of your feet, which causes your head to move backward over your shoulders. This exercise should be repeated frequently during the day in order to retrain yourself in good postural techniques, at least every one to two hours. It is better to do one repetition six or more times per day than to do six repetitions in a row.

Also See:
* Quadratus lumborum (chapter 4)

You may also need to search for trigger points in the *iliopsoas, serratus posterior superior, serratus posterior inferior,* and *latissimus dorsi,* since trigger points in those muscles can either cause similar pain referral patterns or may affect or be affected by *paraspinal* trigger points in some way.

Since trigger points in these muscles don't directly cause chest or abdominal pain, they are not addressed in this book. If you can't relieve your pain with the self-help techniques in this book after six to eight weeks, you may wish to consider whether you need to treat trigger points in these additional muscles, or if you still have perpetuating factors to resolve. Go to the end of this book for other books by the author that provide self-treatment techniques of muscles not covered in this book.

> **Differential Diagnosis:** If you are experiencing pain in the spine, you will need to see a health care provider to rule out herniated discs, spinal stenosis (narrowing of the hole the spinal cord goes through, or of one of the holes the nerves go out through), infections, tumors, cancer, or other more serious problems. Other diagnoses that should be considered are fibromyalgia, organ disease, osteoarthritis, fat lobules, strain of spinal ligaments, retrocecal appendicitis, a dissecting aortic aneurysm or saddle thrombus, kidney stones, torsion of the kidney, pelvic inflammatory disease, endometriosis, ankylosing spondylitis, Paget's disease, leukemia, Hodgkin's disease, prostatitis and seminal vesiculitis, or sacroiliitis. A finding of osteoarthritis in itself may not account for the pain felt, since you can have pain without degenerative changes to the spine, and you can have degenerative changes without pain. Lumbar zygapophysial (facet) joints may refer pain in the same pattern as multifidi muscles.
>
> Vertebrae may be out of alignment and need to be adjusted by a chiropractor or osteopathic physician. Combining acupuncture or massage with adjustments is more helpful, since tight muscles will keep pulling vertebra out of alignment.

Chapter 4: Quadratus Lumborum
(and Iliolumbar Ligament)

In the United States, low back pain causes some degree of work disability in 10-15% of adults per year, costing billions of dollars in sick days, reduced productivity, and health insurance claims. People with disabling low back pain receive more than $3 billion per year just in disability payments. Recognition and treatment of trigger points could reduce these sums substantially. Trigger points in the *quadratus lumborum* muscle are responsible for roughly 30% of sacral-gluteal pain.

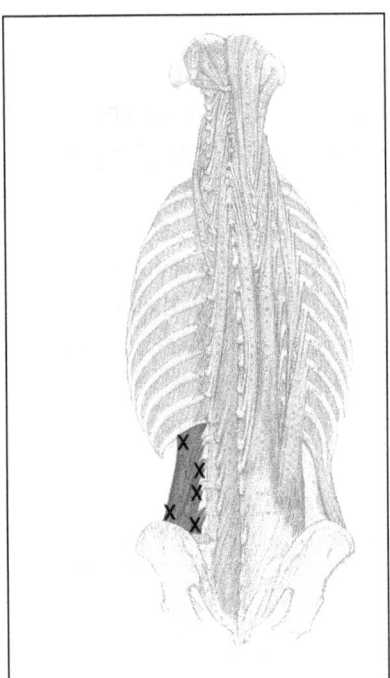
Back view of trunk

Common Symptoms

- depending on the location of the trigger points, pain can be referred to various places in the gluteal area, the sacrum, over the hip joint and surrounding area, and even around the front to the groin area, testis, scrotum, and the lower abdomen (see the pictures for the referral patterns)
- pain is usually deep and aching, but can be sharp or stabbing with movement
- possibly unbearable pain with standing or sitting upright, but you may be able to crawl on your hands and knees
- pain with climbing stairs
- rotating your trunk, or leaning to the opposite side is very painful
- rolling onto your side, getting up, or getting out of a chair may be extremely painful or impossible
- pain can be so intolerable you cannot lie on the affected side
- you may be unable to bear weight on the affected side

- coughing or sneezing can cause unbearable pain temporarily
- range-of-motion can be restricted with bending forward
- pain over the sacroiliac joint (where the sacrum and big pelvic bone join) and greater trochanter (hip joint) can be mistaken for joint dysfunction
- constant pain eventually causes fatigue and probably depression
- a small number of patients may experience a "lightning bolt" of pain down the front of the thigh in a narrow band
- possibly "heaviness of the hips," calf cramping, and burning sensations in the legs and feet
- a "sciatica" type of pain distribution that may be reproduced by pressing on *quadratus lumborum* trigger points and possibly some *gluteus minimus* trigger points ("pseudo-sciatica")

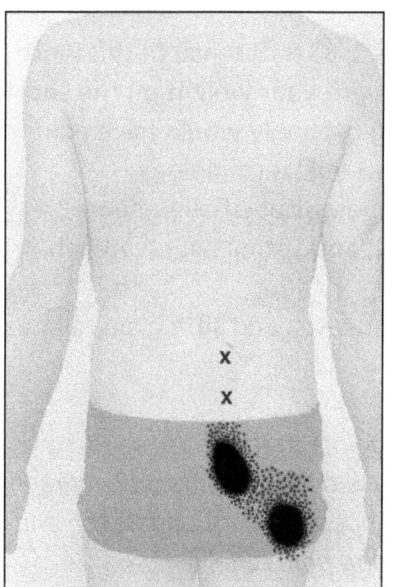
Deep fibers

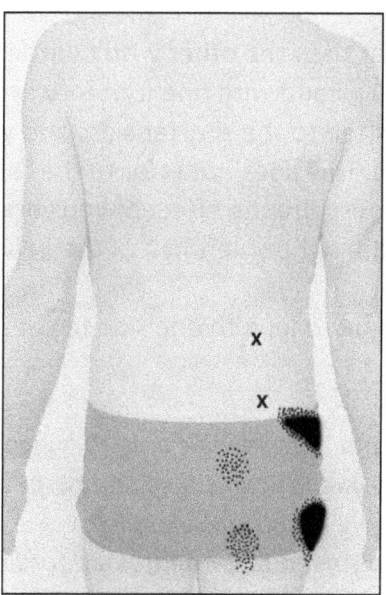
Superficial fibers

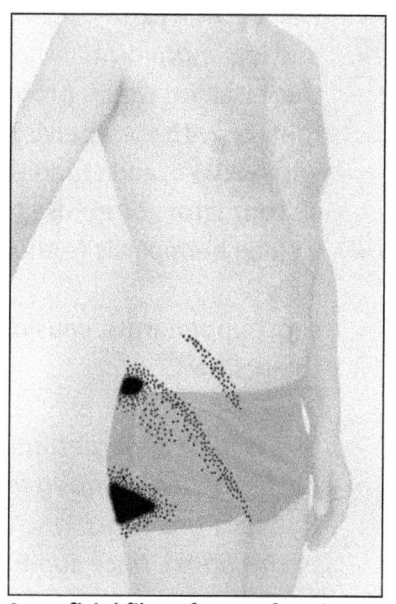
Superficial fibers front referral pattern

- the *iliolumbar ligament* can refer pain locally around the 4th and 5th lumbar vertebrae, but can also cause pain that feels like it is deep in the hip joint, in the groin area, and diffusely over the front of the thigh

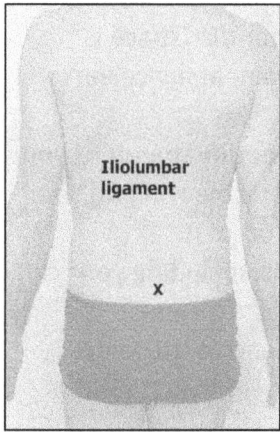

Causes and Perpetuation of Trigger Points

- trauma, such as an auto accident
- awkward movements, such as lifting something heavy, especially when your trunk is rotated at the same time, or trying to rise out of a low chair, car, or bed
- attempting to put on pants, socks, and shoes while standing
- a near fall, where you catch yourself
- a repetitive strain from gardening, washing floors, lifting heavy objects, or walking or running on slanted surfaces such as a beach or road
- leaning forward over a desk, sink, or other work surface
- weak *abdominal* muscles (chapter 11)
- mattresses that are too old or too soft, or sleeping next to someone who is heavier and trying to avoid rolling into them
- walking in a cast
- one leg *anatomically* shorter than the other with as little as 1/8" difference (if this were the case you would probably stand with one foot forward, with your weight on the short foot, or with your pelvis shifted to the shorter side, and you probably would have pain with walking and standing). This does *not* refer to the "short leg" terminology chiropractors often use to describe the effect of vertebrae being out-of-alignment.
- a small hemipelvis (either the right or left half of the pelvis), and sitting aggravates the pain
- short upper arms, causing you to lean to one side to use armrests, and sitting aggravates the pain

This is a list of perpetuating factors specific only to trigger points in this muscle. For a full list of perpetuating factors that can cause and perpetuate trigger points anywhere in the body and which also apply to this muscle, please see "Appendix A" (found at the end of this book), since some may need to be addressed for lasting pain relief.

Helpful Hints

- Some of my patients have assumed their pain in the lumbar region meant they had a kidney infection. Symptoms of a kidney infection include a high fever and chills. **If you are experiencing those symptoms, go to the emergency room immediately**. Otherwise, check for trigger points and see if you can get relief.
- Don't assume that a finding of bone spurs or narrowing of the lumbar disc space is causing the pain, since many people who have these do not have pain, and vice versa. Always assume trigger points are at least a part of the problem.
- You may find relief by lying on your back or side. Using a pillow to modify the tilt of your hips or placing it under your knees may be helpful. If you are comfortable lying on your side, place a pillow in front of your legs and put your upper leg on top of it.
- Always be sure to have proper lumbar support in all sitting locations, including your car.
- Sit while putting on pants, socks, and shoes.
- Avoid any heavy lifting, and if you must lift something, be sure to bend at the knees, keep your torso straight, and keep the object close to your body.

- Stand up straight, rather than bending over sinks and work surfaces. If you must lean over something, keep it brief and support yourself with a free hand.
- When standing up from a chair, slide your butt to the front of the chair, turn your entire body a little sideways, put one foot under the front edge of the chair, then stand with the torso erect so that your thighs take the load. You can use your hands to assist you if necessary. Sit down in the opposite sequence.
- When climbing stairs or a ladder, rotate your entire body 45-degrees and keep your back straight.
- Gardeners should sit on a stool about eight to ten inches high, and take frequent breaks.
- Buy a firm mattress, and replace it every five to seven years. You can put plywood between the box springs and mattress to make it firmer.
- Don't carry a wallet in your back pocket, as this tilts your pelvis when you sit on it.
- Make sure your muscles don't get chilled, especially at night.
- If you must wear a walking cast due to a broken bone, get a shoe for the opposite foot with a sole that matches the height of the bottom of the cast.
- See a specialist for corrective orthotics, and compensating lifts and pads if necessary. If an anatomical leg length inequality is not corrected, it can contribute to osteoarthritis of the hip and lumbar spine. Symptoms from an anatomical leg length inequality may not show up until it is brought on by an acute trauma, such as a car accident. If you use compensating lifts, you must use them all the time, in all shoes, and not go barefoot. (Evaluation of various body asymmetries is discussed in detail in: Janet G. Travell, M.D., and David G. Simons, M.D., *Myofascial Pain and Dysfunction: The Trigger Point Manual, The Lower Extremities vol. 2* (Baltimore: Williams & Wilkins, 1992), pp. 41-63.
- If you are getting an anatomical leg-length inequity corrected with lifts, start with a thin lift and gradually use thicker ones until the proper lift height is reached.
- Armrests can be corrected by taping sponges or towels to the armrests.

Self-Help Techniques

Always do the self-treatment on *both* sides! It is rare that only one side is involved, especially in the lumbar and gluteal muscles. Consider acupuncture for treatment of the *quadratus lumborum*, since needles are better able to penetrate down to the muscle than massage.

Wrapping your hands around the sides of your waist and pressing downward on the top of your pelvis may give enough temporary relief to allow some movement, as may using your thumbs to apply pressure to the muscle itself.

Applying Pressure

Paraspinal Pressure: As part of the quadratus lumborum self-treatment, work on the *paraspinal* muscles (chapter 3), because most of the time those muscles are also involved to some extent.

Quadratus Lumborum Pressure: When you get to the lumbar area, most people have enough of a curve that they might need to move to the floor and use a tennis ball or baseball, but make sure this is not too hard for you (see the general guidelines in chapter 1). Don't use a softball since it is too large. You may use your hand to move the ball, searching for trigger points in the lumbar area. *Do not press your back onto the ball and if you have been diagnosed with bulging or herniated discs, be very careful not to get too close to the spine!*

Iliolumbar Ligament Pressure: The *iliolumbar ligament* is in a small dip between the fifth lumbar vertebra and the rim of your pelvis. It is helpful to locate it with your thumb first. Lying face-up with your knees bent, on a hard surface such as a wood or linoleum floor or on a very thin carpet, use a golf ball and your body weight to give you pressure. If this is not enough pressure, put the calf of the same side on top of the opposite knee. You may also wish to continue down a little further onto the top part of the sacrum, in order to get the S_1 multifidi (see chapter 3 for a picture of the *multifidi* muscles).

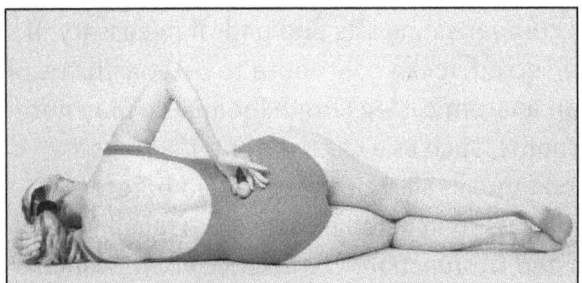
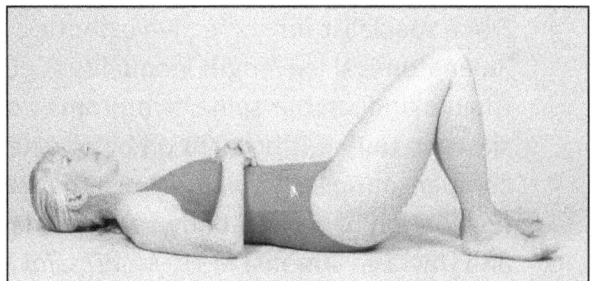

Demonstrating location of iliolumbar ligament

Stretches

Supine Self-Stretch: Lie face-up with your knees bent and with your hands behind your head; if you don't put your hands behind your head, you will not get the stretch. Place one leg over the other knee, and use that leg to gently pull the knee down toward the floor. You should feel the stretch in the lumbar and gluteal areas. Then slip the leg off of the knee, return to neutral position, and repeat on the opposite side. You may repeat this a few times on each side. Follow with the Hip-Hike Stretch below.

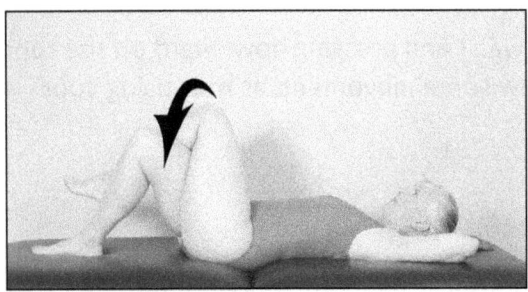
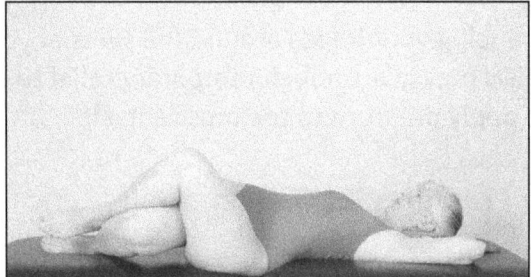

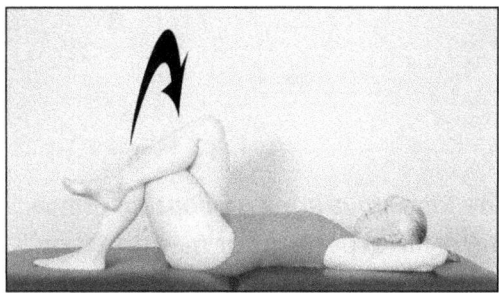 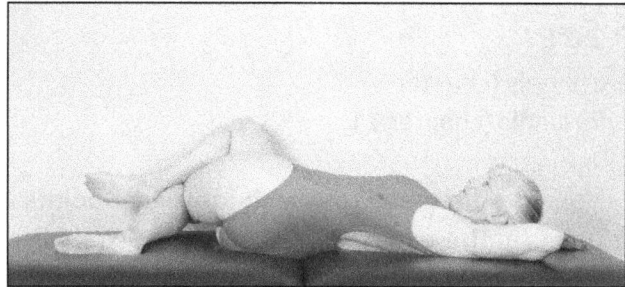

Hip-Hike Stretch: Lie face-up with your legs out straight. Place your hands on your hips, and as you breathe in, stretch one leg down so your pelvis tilts down on that side and you are feeling a stretch in the lumbar area. Exhale as you return to the neutral position. Repeat on the other side.

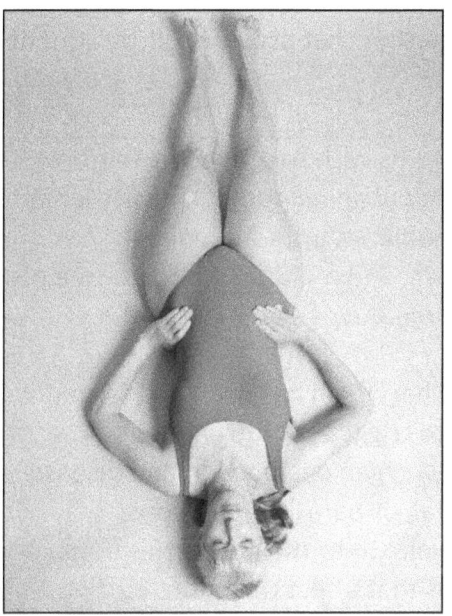 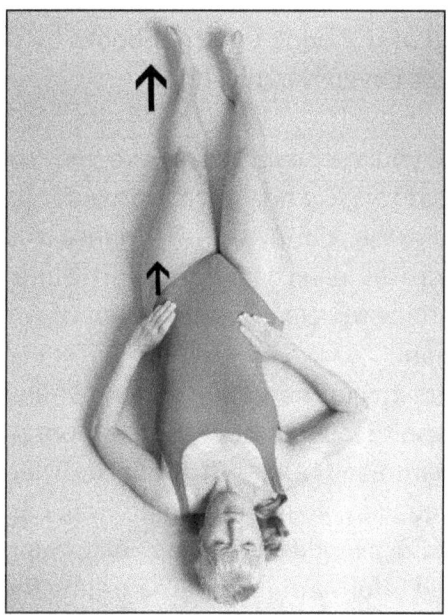

Exercises

Supine Self-Stretch with Resistance: Once trigger points have been inactivated for a few weeks and are no longer causing referred pain, during the Supine Self-Stretch you may briefly apply resistance to provide an additional stretch. While you are using the left leg to stretch the right side, briefly use the right knee to push up against the left leg, then relax, taking up the slack in the stretch, and repeat. Do the same on the opposite side.

Also See:
*   Paraspinals (chapter 3)
*   Abdominals (chapter 11)

You may also need to search for trigger points in the *latissimus dorsi* or *iliopsoas*, since trigger points in these muscles can either cause similar pain referral patterns or may affect or be affected by *quadratus lumborum* trigger points in some way. You may need to check the *gluteus medius*, since trigger points in that muscle can activate *quadratus lumborum* trigger points. Trigger points in the *gluteus medius* and *gluteus minimus* muscles can cause weakness in the *quadratus lumborum*. Since trigger points in these muscles don't directly cause chest or abdominal pain, they are not addressed in this book. If you can't relieve your pain with the self-help techniques in this book after six to eight weeks, you may wish to consider whether you need to treat trigger points in these additional muscles, or if you still have perpetuating factors to resolve. Go to the end of this book for other books by the author that provide self-treatment techniques of muscles not covered in this book.

> **Differential Diagnosis:** If you are unable to relieve your symptoms with trigger point self-help techniques, you may need to see a health care provider to rule out spinal tumors, myasthenia gravis, gallstones, liver disease, kidney stones, urinary tract problems, intra-abdominal infections, intestinal parasites, diverticulitis, an aortic aneurysm, and multiple sclerosis. See a chiropractor or osteopathic physician for evaluation of vertebrae out of alignment and sacroiliac joint subluxation.
>
> Be sure to address any perpetuating factors when low back pain has persisted for more than a few weeks or doesn't respond more than temporarily to trigger point treatment. Particularly examine vitamin and other nutritional deficiencies, organ dysfunction and disease especially thyroid inadequacies, acute or chronic viral, bacterial, or parasitic infections, emotional factors, or active allergies with a high histamine level. Go to the end of this book, "Appendix A" for detailed information on perpetuating factors that affect the entire body.

Chapter 5: Pectoralis Major & Subclavius

This muscle covers much of the chest, and can cause shoulders to be rounded forward in a slumped-looking posture. *Pectoralis major* trigger points can mimic the symptoms of a heart attack, but can also be caused by a heart attack, so heart and lung problems must be ruled out before assuming it is trigger points only.

The *pectoralis major* may get involved in a "frozen shoulder" syndrome.

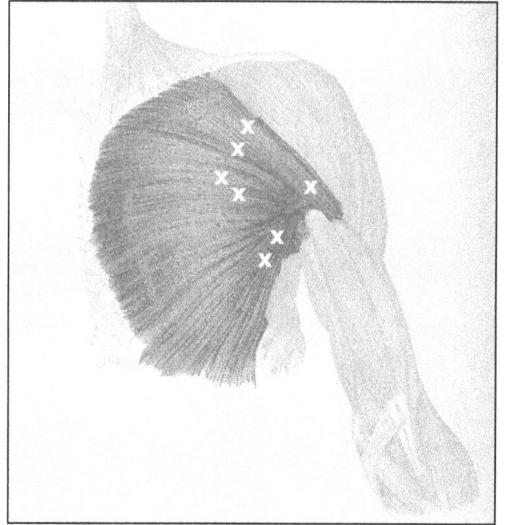
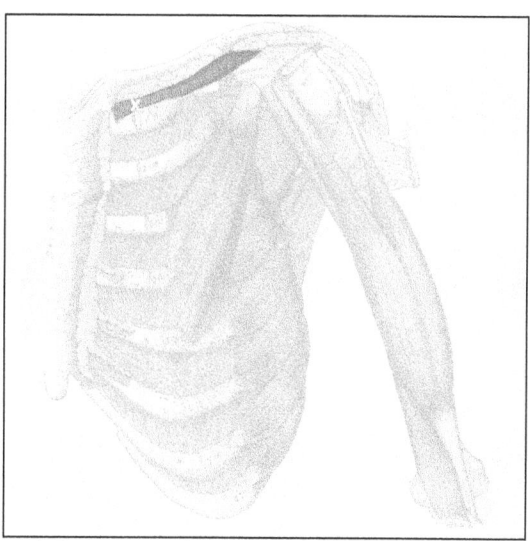

Pectoralis Major muscle, chest area   **Subclavius muscle, under collarbone**

Common Symptoms

- referred pain in the chest, shoulder, breast, and down the inner arm, possibly all the way into the hand
- mid-back pain caused by shortening of the *pectoralis* muscles, even if the *pectoralis* trigger points are latent (not causing referred pain of their own)
- activated or perpetuated trigger points in the *sternocleidomastoid* muscle (chapter 8), along with the subsequent symptoms of those trigger points
- restricted range-of-motion
- chest constriction
- pain may disturb sleep
- breast tenderness, hypersensitivity of the nipple, and/or irritation by clothing on the breast
- there may be a feeling of congestion in the breast, a slight enlargement, and a "doughy" feeling caused by impaired lymph drainage
- a sudden, extreme sharp pain during a sudden overload to the muscle may indicate a torn muscle

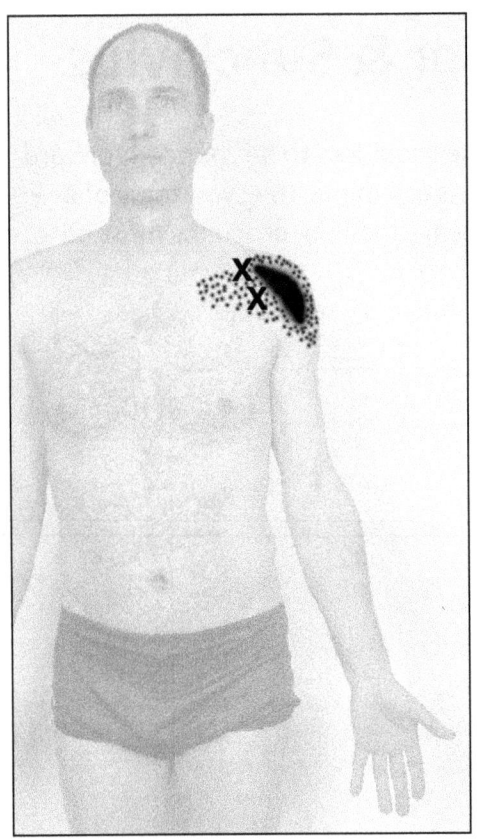
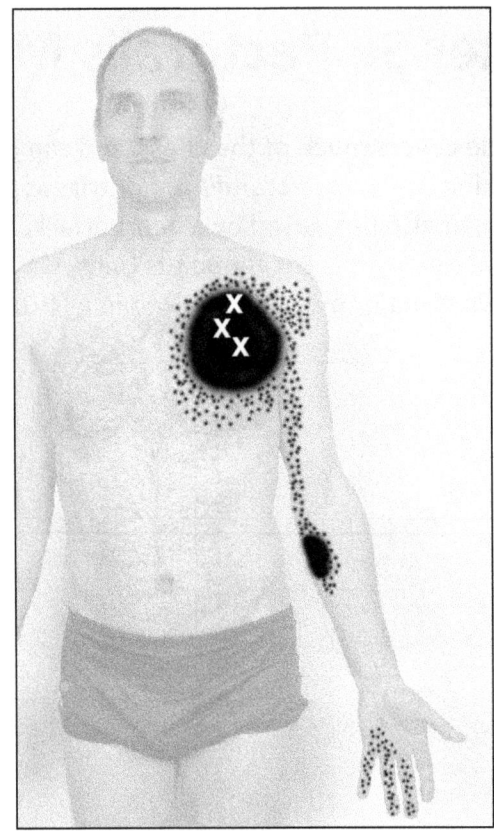
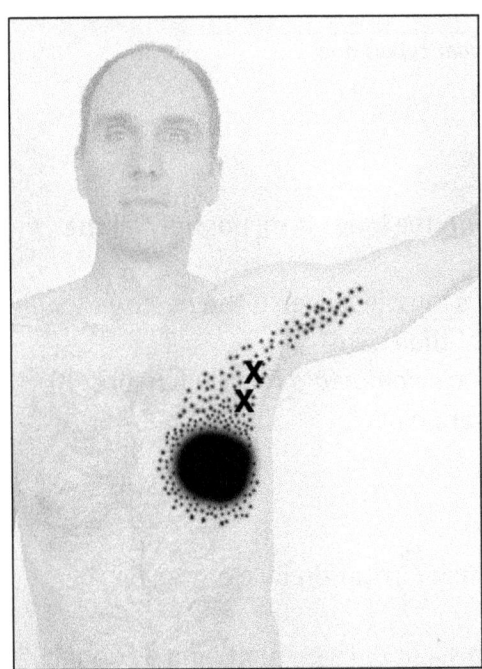
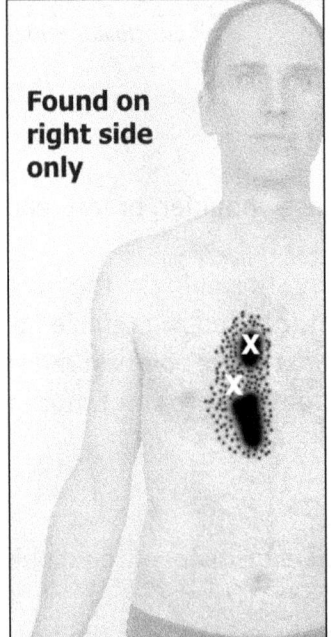

Various pectoralis major referral patterns

- ectopic cardiac arrhythmias such as supraventricular tachycardia, supraventricular premature contractions, or ventricular premature contractions can be caused by a particular point on the right side of the trunk only, between the 5th and 6th rib, about 1-2" to the left of the nipple

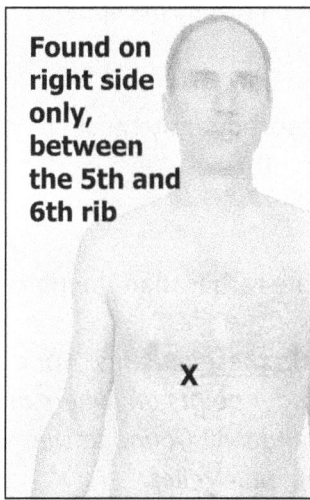

- the *subclavius* can cause pain under the collar bone, down the front upper arm, down the outside of the lower arm, and into the thumb, index, and middle fingers

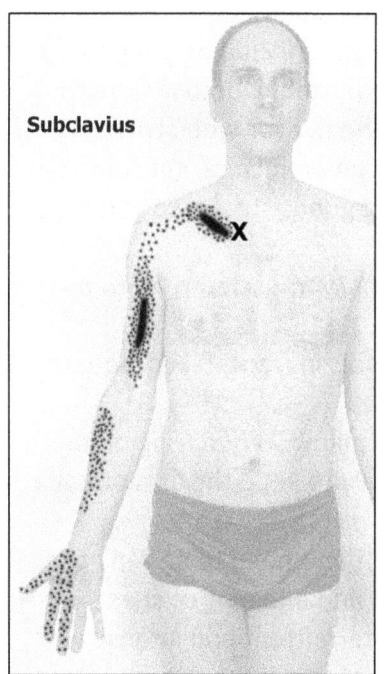 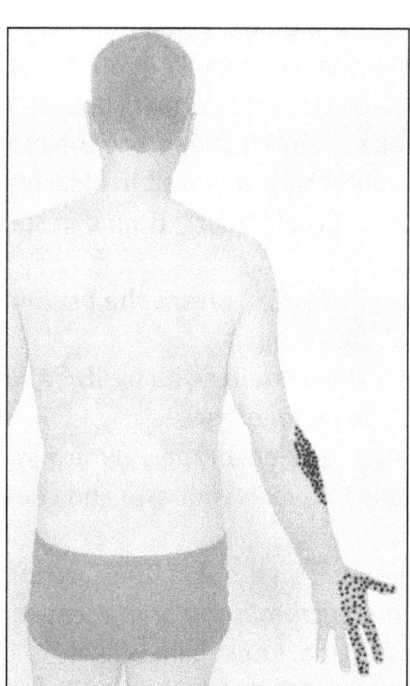

Subclavius front referral pattern   *Subclavius back referral pattern*

Causes and Perpetuation of Trigger Points

- poor posture while sitting, or slouching while standing, allowing your shoulders to round forward.
- heavy lifting, especially when reaching out
- overuse by bringing your arms together repetitively, as in using a pair of bush clippers
- sustained lifting in front, as with a chainsaw
- your arm being immobilized in a cast or sling
- constant anxiety, probably resulting in holding your breath and subsequently causing trigger points to form
- exposure to cold air when the muscles are fatigued
- a heart attack
- open heart surgery where the incision was through the breastbone rather than the ribs

This is a list of perpetuating factors specific only to trigger points in these muscles. For a full list of perpetuating factors that can cause and perpetuate trigger points anywhere in the body and which also apply to these muscles, please see "Appendix A" (found at the end of this book), since some may need to be addressed for lasting pain relief.

Helpful Hints

- Get a good pair of custom orthotics that will shift your weight slightly to the balls of your feet. This will shift your head back over your shoulders and restore normal cervical and lumbar curves, bring the shoulders back, and open up the chest.
- Get a chair with a good lumbar support. For your car or any seat (including your couch at home) that doesn't have adequate lumbar support, get a portable lumbar support. You may wish to even take a lumbar support to the movie theatre, or when traveling for use on airplanes and in rental cars. If you sit in bleachers or go on picnics, get some type of back support like a **Crazy Creek Chair**™ (found in sporting goods stores) so you have at least some kind of support.
- Crossing your arms in front of you shortens the *pectoralis major* muscle, so try to use armrests at the height of your elbows.
- If you must perform work that requires you to lift or hold tools in front, take frequent breaks, or avoid the activity all together.
- When lying on your unaffected side, drape your arm over a pillow. When lying on the affected side, tuck a pillow between your arm and chest/belly to keep the arm out at a 90-degree angle.
- If your bras leave indentations on the skin, they are too tight and need to be replaced.
- Active trigger points in the *pectoralis major* may cause pain and a feeling of chest constriction that mimics angina. Chest pain is likely to be intermittent and intense with moving the upper arm, and there may also possibly be pain at rest if the trigger points are very active. Pain can disturb sleep. Remember that angina and trigger points can exist concurrently, so you will *still need to undergo cardiac function tests even if you are able to relieve pain with trigger point self-help techniques*. Non-cardiac pain may induce transient T-wave changes in the electrocardiogram, so further tests may be needed. Even with heart disease, pain from trigger points may reflexively diminish the size of the

coronary arteries thereby further increasing myocardial ischemia, so relief of trigger points can increase cardiac circulation in addition to increasing comfort.
- Shortening of the *subclavius* muscle by trigger points can contribute to vascular thoracic outlet syndrome by causing the clavicle to compress the subclavian artery and vein against the first rib.

Self-Help Techniques

Applying Pressure

Pectoralis Pressure: Lie face-down with the arm on the side you are treating next to your side. Place a ball above the breast area and be sure to work all the way out to the armpit. You may need to shift your weight a little to the side you are working on as you work out toward the armpit. You may also try hanging your arm over the side of the bed, if it is high enough to allow your arm to dangle. If you are large-breasted, you may find it easier to place the ball on the end of a couch arm or wall and lean into it, but be sure to keep your arm relaxed.

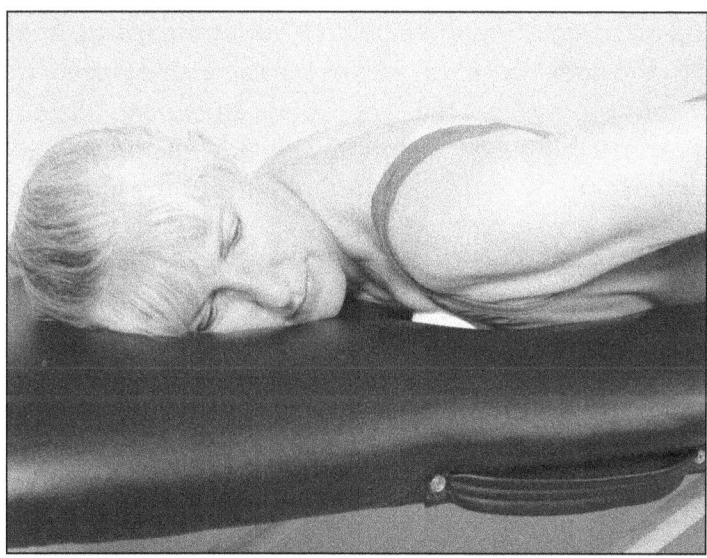
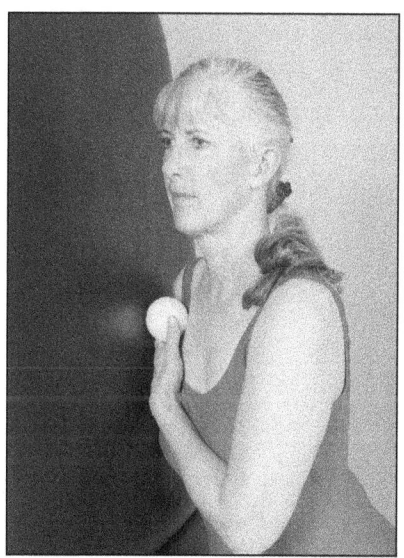

Subclavius Pressure: Much of the *subclavius* muscle is under the collarbone, so you must lean forward, allowing your arm to dangle, which moves the collarbone away from the trunk. With the opposite hand, press under the collarbone with your fingers, especially working closer to the breastbone.

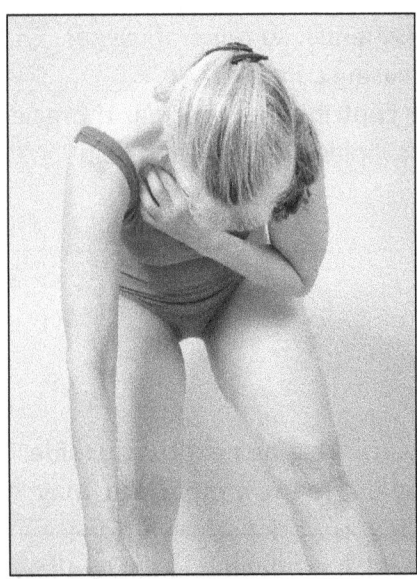

Stretches

Pectoralis Stretch: Stand in a doorway and place your forearm along the door frame, including your elbow, with your upper arm parallel to the floor. With the foot of the same side placed about one step forward, rotate your body gently away from the side you are stretching. Move your forearm up to about a 45° angle and repeat. Bring the forearm down below the first position and repeat. The different forearm positions will stretch different parts of the muscle.

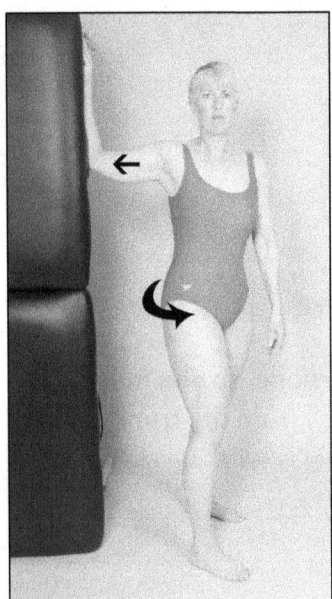

Position 1

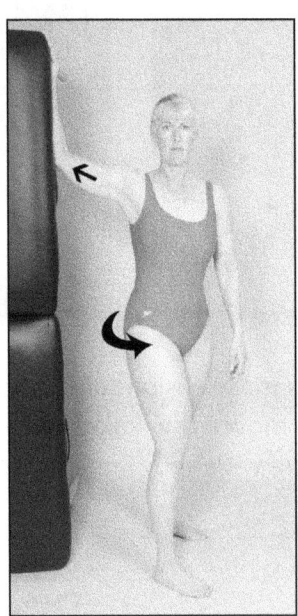

Position 2

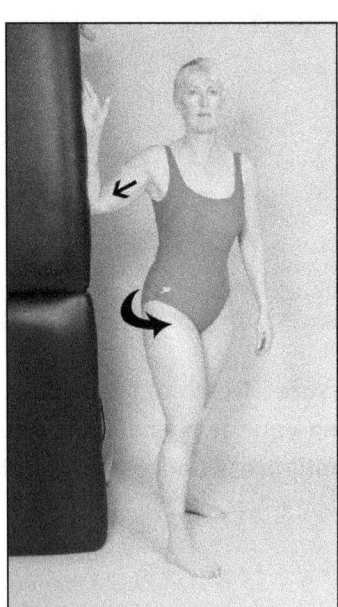

Position 3

Also See:
* Scalene (chapter 9)
* Paraspinal (chapter 3)
* Sternalis (chapter 7)
* Sternocleidomastoid (chapter 8)

If you have pectoralis major trigger points, you may also need to work on the anterior *deltoid, coracobrachialis, scalenes* (chapter 9), *trapezius*, and *rhomboid* muscles, since they will tend to develop satellite trigger points. The *trapezius* and *rhomboid* muscles may become painful after relieving *pectoralis major* trigger points, so you may need to perform self-treatment on those muscles after the *pectoralis major* muscle.

You may also need to search for trigger points in the *sternocleidomastoid (chapter 8)*, *sternalis (chapter 7)*, and/or *serratus anterior*, since trigger points in those muscles also tend to develop satellite trigger points.

If you have a frozen shoulder from pectoralis muscle involvement, you may also need to work on the *subscapularis, infraspinatus, teres minor*, and posterior *deltoid* muscles.

If you have been diagnosed with thoracic outlet syndrome, you may also need to check the *latissimus dorsi, teres major, scalenes* (chapter 9), and *subscapularis* muscles, since trigger points there may mimic thoracic outlet syndrome.

Since trigger points in the *deltoid, coracobrachialis, trapezius, rhomboid, serratus anterior, subscapularis, infraspinatus, teres minor, latissimus dorsi, teres major*, and *subscapularis* muscles don't directly cause chest or abdominal pain, they are not addressed in this book. If you can't relieve your pain with the self-help techniques in this book after six to eight weeks, you may wish to consider whether you need to treat trigger points in these additional muscles, or if you still have perpetuating factors to resolve. Go to the end of this book for other books by the author that provide self-treatment techniques of muscles not covered in this book.

> **Differential Diagnosis:** If you are unable to relieve your symptoms with trigger point self-help techniques, you may need to see a health care provider to rule out angina, muscle tears, bicipital tendinitis, supraspinatus tendinitis, subacromial bursitis, medial epicondylitis, lateral epicondylitis, C_5 to C_8 nerve root irritation, intercostal neuritis or radiculopathy, irritation of the bronchi, pleura, or esophagus, a hiatal hernia with reflux, distention of the stomach by gas, mediastinal emphysema, gaseous distention of the splenic flexure of the colon, coronary insufficiency, fibromyalgia, and lung cancer. A sudden, extreme sharp pain during a sudden overload of the muscle may indicate a torn muscle. Skeletal diagnoses that need to be considered include chest wall syndrome, Tietze's syndrome, costochondritis, hypersensitive xiphoid process syndrome, precordial catch syndrome, slipping rib syndrome, and rib-tip syndrome, though many of these may be due either entirely or in part to trigger points.

Chapter 6: Pectoralis Minor

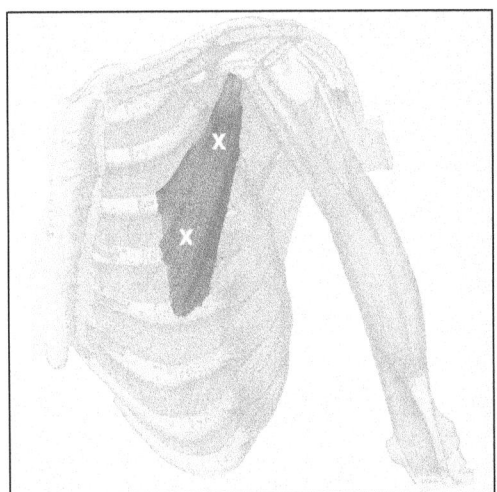

View of front of chest, under pectoralis major muscle

Common Symptoms

- referred pain mainly over the front of the shoulder, and sometimes over the chest and/or down the inside of the arm into the middle, ring, and little fingers
- shoulders that are rounded forward
- range-of-motion restricted when reaching forward and upward, or reaching backward with the arm at shoulder level
- symptoms may mimic angina
- difficulty in taking a deep breath
- a *pectoralis minor* entrapment (pinching the axillary artery and the brachial plexus nerve) can be mis-diagnosed as carpal tunnel syndrome, and will not be resolved by carpal tunnel surgery
- entrapment of the brachial plexus nerve by the *pectoralis minor* muscle causes numbness and uncomfortable sensations of the ring and little fingers, back of the hand, outside of the forearm, and palm side of the thumb, index and middle fingers
- shortening of the *pectoralis minor* muscle fibers as a result of trigger points may lead to "coracoid pressure syndrome," arm pain, and weakness of muscles in the mid-back in the areas of the lower portion of the *trapezius* and *rhomboid* muscles

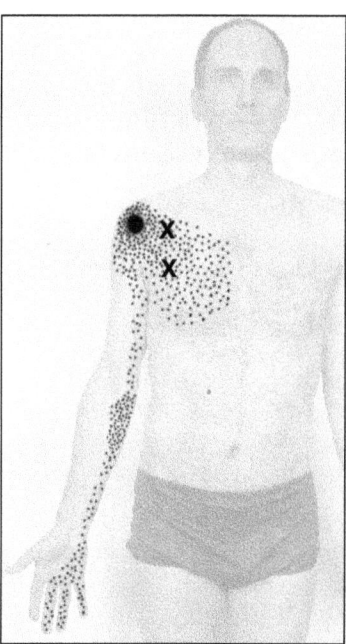

Causes and Perpetuation of Trigger Points
- poor posture, especially when seated
- wearing a daypack or backpack without a chest strap, allowing the shoulder straps to compress the muscle
- gardening
- *scalene* (chapter 9) or *pectoralis major* (chapter 5) trigger points
- weakness of the lower portion of the *trapezius* muscle
- trauma, such as fractured ribs or firing a rifle with the butt on the chest instead of the front of the shoulder
- using crutches
- coughing and/or improper breathing
- a whiplash injury
- angina pain
- open-heart surgery that was conducted through the breastbone (sternum) rather than the ribs

This is a list of perpetuating factors specific only to trigger points in this muscle. For a full list of perpetuating factors that can cause and perpetuate trigger points anywhere in the body and which also apply to this muscle, please see "Appendix A" (found at the end of this book), since some may need to be addressed for lasting pain relief.

Helpful Hints
- Modify or replace your mis-fitting furniture. Your knees should fit under your desk, and the chair needs to be close enough that you can lean against your backrest. Your elbows should rest on either your work surface or armrests at the same height. Your elbows and forearms should rest evenly on the armrests. Your computer screen should be directly in

front of you, and the copy attached to the side of the screen, so that you may look directly forward as much as possible.
- Use crutches properly by supporting your weight on your hands, not your armpits.
- Be sure to use a pack with proper shoulder padding and a chest strap to distribute weight away from the armpit area.
- Learn to breathe properly; see chapter 9.
- Avoid bras that compress the *pectoralis minor* muscle. Try to find one with a wider shoulder strap or a padded strap.

Self-Help Techniques

Check for trigger points in the *pectoralis major* (chapter 5) and *scalene* (chapter 9) muscles, since they will keep trigger points in the *pectoralis minor* activated.

Applying Pressure

Pectoralis Major Pressure: The *pectoralis major* pressure (chapter 5) will also treat the underlying *pectoralis minor* muscle.

Stretches

Pectoralis Stretch: See chapter 5.

Also See:
* Pectoralis major (chapter 5)
* Scalene (chapter 9)
* Sternocleidomastoid (chapter 8)
* Sternalis (chapter 7)

You may need to check the *deltoid* for satellite trigger points after treating the *pectoralis* muscles. Since trigger points in this muscle don't directly cause chest or abdominal pain, it is not addressed in this book. If you can't relieve your pain with the self-help techniques in this book after six to eight weeks, you may wish to consider whether you need to treat trigger points in this additional muscle, or if you still have perpetuating factors to resolve. Go to the end of this book for other books by the author that provide self-treatment techniques of muscles not covered in this book.

Differential Diagnosis: If you are unable to relieve your symptoms with trigger point self-help techniques, you may need to see a health care provider to rule out *true* thoracic outlet syndrome, C_7 and C_8 nerve root irritation, supraspinatus tendonitis, bicipital tendonitis, and medial epicondylitis. You may need to see a chiropractor or osteopathic physician to be evaluated for elevation of the third, fourth, and fifth ribs.

Chapter 7: Sternalis

Only about 5% of people have this muscle, and it may possibly be found on only one side.

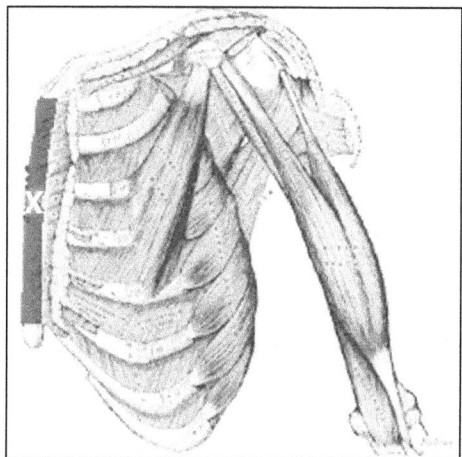

Front view of chest

Common Symptoms

- a deep intense ache under the sternum, or "breastbone," that may also extend across the upper chest, into the front of your shoulder, and down the inner upper arm to your elbow, or on the left side, past your elbow
- symptoms may be mistaken for a heart attack or angina
- trigger points are more common in the upper two-thirds of the muscle, and on the left side
- a trigger point located around the top of the muscle may be a source of a dry, hacking cough

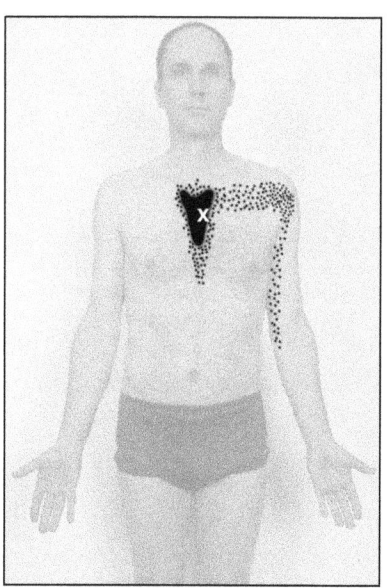

Causes and Perpetuation of Trigger Points
- an acute heart attack or angina
- trigger points may develop as satellite trigger points to the *sternocleidomastoid* muscle (chapter 8)
- a direct trauma to the area

This is a list of perpetuating factors specific only to trigger points in this muscle. For a full list of perpetuating factors that can cause and perpetuate trigger points anywhere in the body and which also apply to this muscle, please see "Appendix A" (found at the end of this book), since some may need to be addressed for lasting pain relief.

Helpful Hints
- Acupuncture is also helpful for treating pain in this area, and pain that feels deep to the rib cage.

Self-Help Techniques

Be sure to check the *sternocleidomastoid* muscle (chapter 8) first for trigger points that may be perpetuating *sternalis* trigger points. Usually trigger points are also found in the *pectoralis major* muscle (chapter 5).

Applying Pressure

Sternalis Pressure: Trigger points are more common in the upper two-thirds of the muscle, and on the left side of the breastbone (sternum). Use the middle three fingers of one hand to apply pressure. If you need more pressure, place your opposite hand over the one you are using to apply pressure. Follow the treatment with moist heat.

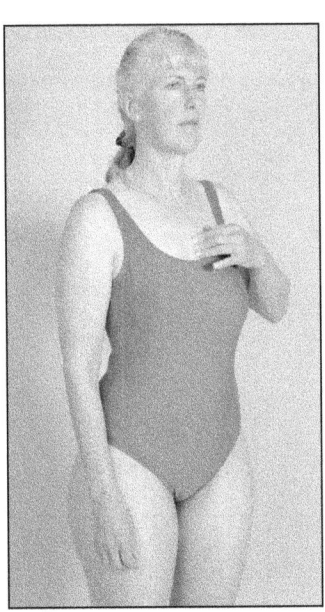

Also See:
* Sternocleidomastoid (chapter 8)
* Pectoralis major (chapter 5)

Differential Diagnosis: *Sternalis* pain may be diagnosed as costochondritis, but you should check for trigger points. If you are unable to relieve trigger points with the self-help, you may need to see a health care provider to check for possible gastroesophageal reflux, esophagitis, and C_7 nerve root irritation.

Chapter 8: Sternocleidomastoid

There are two parts of the *sternocleidomastoid* muscle -- the sternal and clavicular divisions. Each part has different referral patterns and different common symptoms.

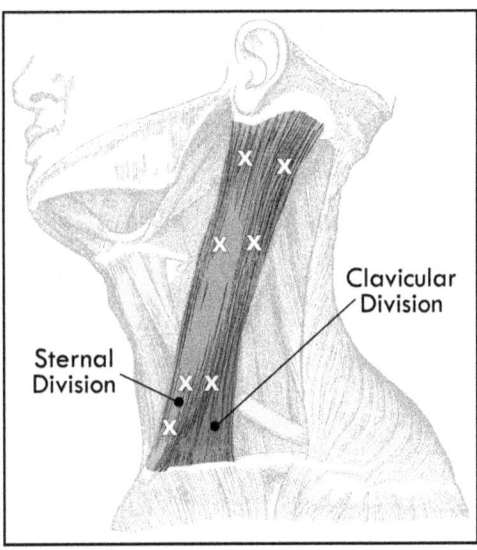

Common Symptoms
- a "tension" headache
- the muscles may be sore to the touch
- a persistent, dry, tickling cough
- entrapment of cranial nerve XI by the *sternocleidomastoid* may cause partial paralysis of the *trapezius* on the same side

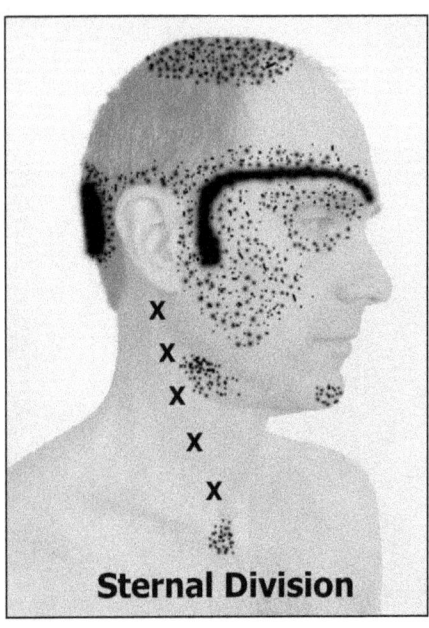
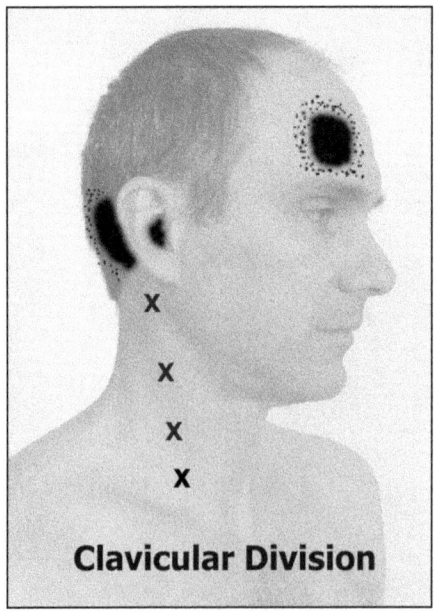

Sternal Division
- referred symptoms to the top of your head, the back of your head, your cheek, and/or over the top of or behind your eye
- sinus congestion on the affected side
- a chronic sore throat (due to referred pain to the throat and back of the tongue when swallowing, rather than infection)
- profuse tearing of your eye
- reddening of the eye whites and the insides of your lids
- visual disturbances, including blurring of vision and/or dimming of perceived light intensity
- a drooping upper eyelid
- eye lid twitching
- occasionally one-sided deafness or a crackling sound in the ear

Clavicular Division
- headaches on your forehead, possibly across the whole forehead rather than just on one side
- earaches (deep pain)
- referred symptoms to your eyes and sinuses (self-work can help clear the sinuses)
- pain in your cheek and molar teeth on the affected side
- dizziness and disturbed balance (disorientation), or vertigo (a spinning sensation), especially when changing position
- nausea and loss of appetite
- trigger points may contribute to seasickness or car sickness
- veering into doorjambs or objects on the affected side
- an inability to drive a car without veering to the side
- an inability to gage differences in weights held in your hands
- sweating, blanching, and a cool sensation on the forehead

Causes and Perpetuation of Trigger Points
- a pillow that is too high
- overhead work (i.e., painting a ceiling) or looking up for long periods of time
- reading in bed with a light off to the side
- constantly tilting your head to avoid light reflection on glasses or contacts, or to improve hearing
- any profession or activity that requires you to tilt your head back or turn it to the side for long periods
- a necktie or collar that is too tight
- a tight *pectoralis major* muscle pulling down and forward on the collar bone (chapter 5)
- swimming (turning your head to breathe)
- horseback riding and horse-handling
- head-forward posture
- whiplash (a car accident, falling on your head, or any sudden jerk of your head)
- a chronic cough

- breathing improperly
- "hangover headaches" may be the result of alcohol stimulating trigger points in the *sternocleidomastoid*
- leakage of cerebrospinal fluid following a spinal tap may activate *sternocleidomastoid* points, and subsequently cause a chronic headache that may last from weeks to years
- chronic infection, such as sinusitis, a dental abscess, or oral herpes (cold sores)
- acute infections, such as the common cold or flu, can activate latent trigger points
- a severe deformity or injury that restricts upper body movement, forcing your neck to overcompensate to keep balance
- an unequal leg length or hemi-pelvis size (either the right or left half of the pelvis)
- severe scoliosis (a curved and/or rotated spine)

This is a list of perpetuating factors specific only to trigger points in this muscle. For a full list of perpetuating factors that can cause and perpetuate trigger points anywhere in the body and which also apply to this muscle, please see "Appendix A" (found at the end of this book), since some may need to be addressed for lasting pain relief.

Helpful Hints

- When lying down, do not get up by leading with your head. First roll onto your side or front, then use your arms to get you started. When turning over in bed at night, roll your head on the pillow, rather than lifting your head to turn. When sleeping, try to keep your head facing in the same direction as your torso, rather than turned to the side. Your pillow should comfortably support the weight of your head, and not be too high or too low. Do not use a foam pillow, as this muscle is especially vulnerable to the jiggling and vibration caused by a foam pillow.
- Reading in bed is not a good idea, but if you are not willing to give this up, then make sure your light is located directly overhead, either on the headboard or ceiling. Keep your head facing in the same direction as your torso, rather than turned to the side. A comfortable chair next to the bed, with appropriate lighting, is even better.
- Get a headset or speaker for your phone.
- If you type, the copy should be as close as possible to the computer screen, so that you are not rotating your head to the side for long periods.
- Avoid head rests that push your head forward. A lumbar pillow may help restore normal lumbar and cervical curves.
- Avoid any overhead work that requires you to bend your head backward.
- *Do not do head-rolling exercises!!* In particular, do not bend or roll your head backwards.
- Your finger should fit comfortably inside your shirt collar, even when your head is turned. Make sure your tie is not too tight.
- If you are a swimmer, avoid the crawl stroke, or any stroke that requires you to turn your head to one side to breathe.
- Nearsightedness needs to be corrected, because you may be holding your head forward to read and see.

- Restoration of proper posture, especially head positioning, is critical to treating trigger points since head-forward posture can both cause and perpetuate trigger points. Head-forward posture can be aggravated while sitting in a car, at a desk, in front of a computer, or while eating dinner or watching TV. Using a good lumbar support everywhere you sit will help correct poor sitting posture. Orthotic inserts in your shoes may improve your standing posture. See chapter 3 for postural re-training.
- If you have a body asymmetry, such as a small hemipelvis (either the right or left half of the pelvis) or an anatomically shorter leg or upper arm, see a specialist to get compensating lifts or pads (this does *not* refer to the "short leg" terminology chiropractors often use to describe the effect of vertebrae being out-of-alignment). Chiropractic adjustments, acupuncture, and massage can help reduce scoliosis.
- Chronic infections must be eliminated or controlled as much as possible (see "Appendix A"). You will probably need to work on your *sternocleidomastoid* muscles after illnesses such as a cold, flu, or facial herpes outbreak (cold sores).
- The chronic cough from asthma and emphysema can aggravate trigger points, as can breathing improperly. See chapter 9 to learn proper breathing techniques.
- Be sure to check the *pectoralis major* muscle (chapter 5) to make sure it is not causing the *sternocleidomastoid* to be pulled tight. If you are doing the *pectoralis* in-doorway stretch, be sure to bring your head back over your shoulders and look straight forward.

Self-Help Techniques

Applying Pressure

Sternocleidomastoid Pressure: It is best to do this self-treatment lying down, but you can do it sitting up, which comes in handy at work. Tilt your head just a little toward the side you are working on (bringing the ear closer to the shoulder) and then rotate your head slightly *away* from that side.

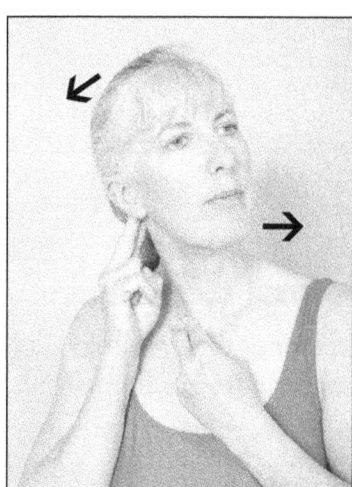

To work the lower half of the muscle, grasp *both* parts of the muscle with your hand of the same side (i.e. the right hand grasps the right sternocleidomastoid), but *don't dig your fingers deep into the neck!* Pinch and pull at the same time, holding each tender spot for eight seconds to one minute.

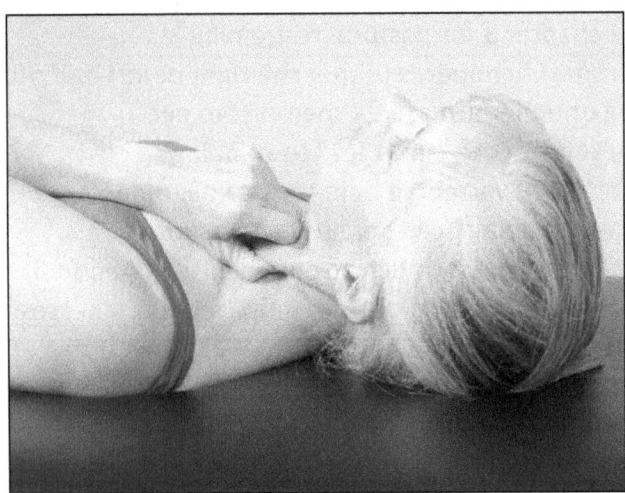

To work the upper half of the muscle, switch hands (i.e. the left hand grasps the right sternocleidomastoid) and pull the muscle outward in the middle. Then use the hand of the same side to work your way up to the attachment behind the ear.

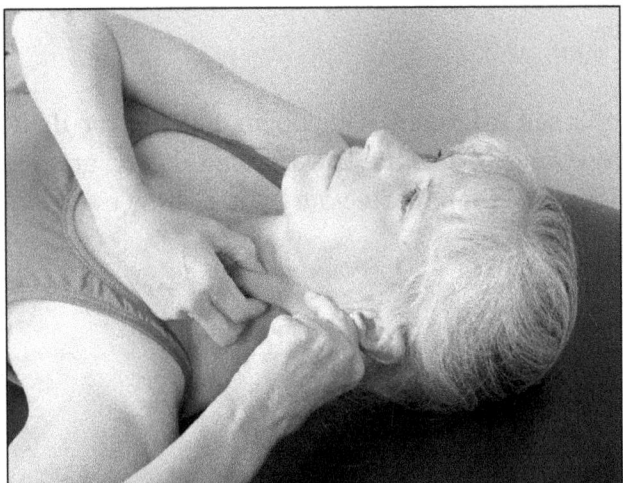

For most people, this is the tightest part, but also the most critical to work on. If your sternocleidomastoid is particularly tight, it may be hard to get a hold of it at first, but after you have worked on it a few times, it should become easier to grasp. Remember that you may have to work this muscle again after an illness, because sternocleidomastoid trigger points will likely be reaggravated.

Copyright © 2024 Valerie DeLaune, LAc

Stretches

Side-Bending Neck Stretch: See chapter 9.

Also See:
* Scalene (chapter 9)
* Sternalis (chapter 7, satellite trigger points)
* Pectoralis major (chapter 5)

If you have *sternocleidomastoid* trigger points, you may need to do the self-help techniques for the posterior neck muscles. These are found in chapter 3.

You may also need to work on the *trapezius, masseter* (satellite trigger points), *platysma, levator scapulae, temporalis* (satellite trigger points), and *platysma* muscles (satellite trigger points) muscles.

Since trigger points in these muscles don't directly cause chest or abdominal pain, they are not addressed in this book. If you can't relieve your pain with the self-help techniques in this book after six to eight weeks, you may wish to consider whether you need to treat trigger points in these additional muscles, or if you still have perpetuating factors to resolve. Go to the end of this book for other books by the author that provide self-treatment techniques of muscles not covered in this book.

Differential Diagnosis: If you are unable to relieve your symptoms with trigger point self-help techniques, you may need to see a health care provider to rule out non-trigger point related headaches, atypical facial neuralgia, trigeminal neuralgia, dizziness caused by problems within the ears, Ménière's disease, tic douloureux, arthritis of the sternoclavicular joint, and wryneck (where the neck is twisted to the side due to muscle spasming).

Chapter 9: Scalenes

Scalene trigger points are a major contributor to back, shoulder, and arm pain, and are commonly overlooked. They also contribute to headaches when combined with trigger points in neck and chewing muscles. They can also refer to the chest.

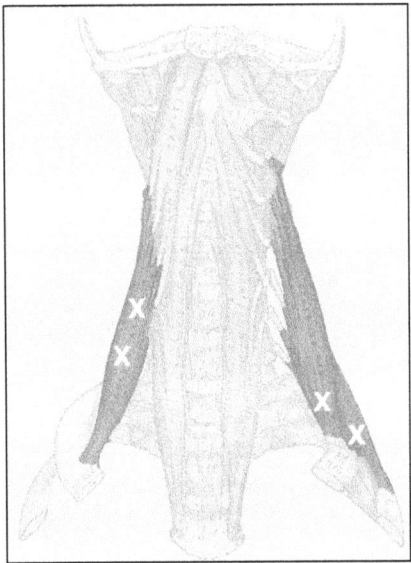

Front View of Neck

Common Symptoms

- pain referred to the chest, mid-back, and/or over the outside, back, and front of the arm and into the wrist and hand
- pain that disturbs sleep, but is relieved by sleeping sitting or propped up
- pain on the left side may be mistaken for angina
- perceived numbness of the thumb (but not actual), and tingling
- dropping items unexpectedly
- possibly finger stiffness
- minimal restriction of range-of-motion when rotating your head, but greater restriction when bending it to the side
- you may be able to reproduce pain by turning your head to the side and then putting your chin down toward your shoulder
- you may be able to relieve pain by putting the back of your forearm across your forehead and moving your elbow forward (which moves the collarbone away from the *scalene* muscle)
- a tight *scalene* muscle may elevate the first rib, leading to compressed nerves, arteries, veins, and lymph ducts, causing numbness, tingling, and loss of sensation in the 4th and 5th fingers and side of the hand, and stiffness and swelling in the fingers and back of your hand which is worse in the morning
- phantom limb pain in amputees

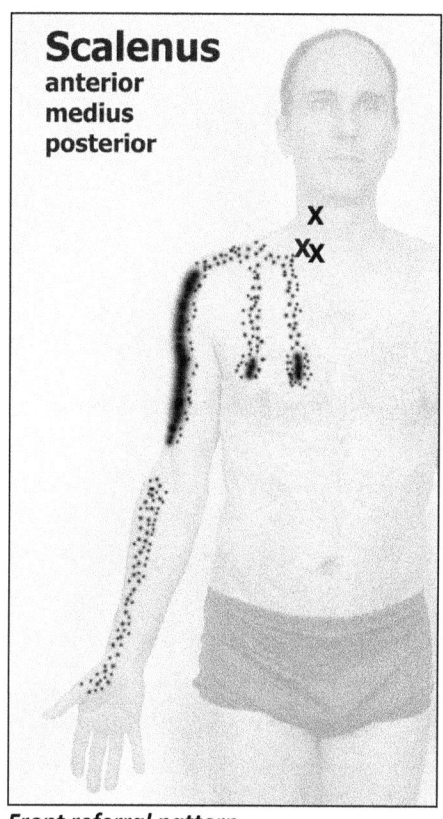
Front referral pattern

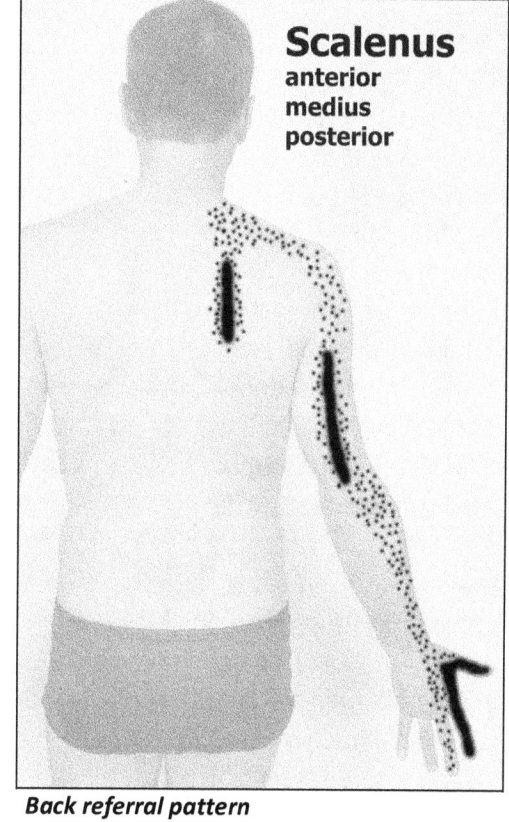
Back referral pattern

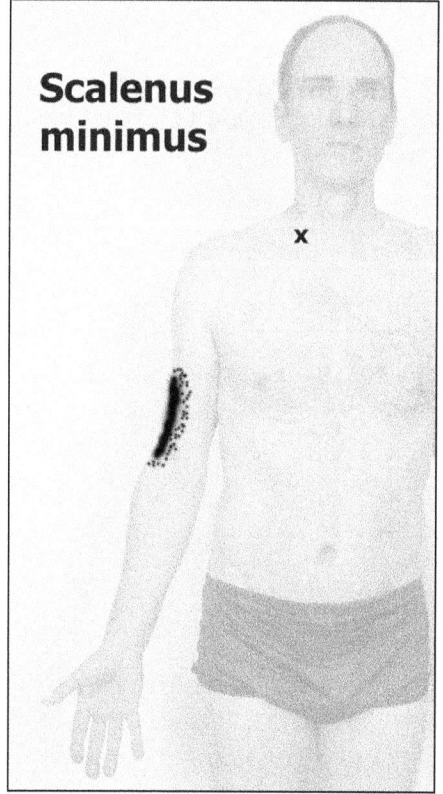
Front referral pattern

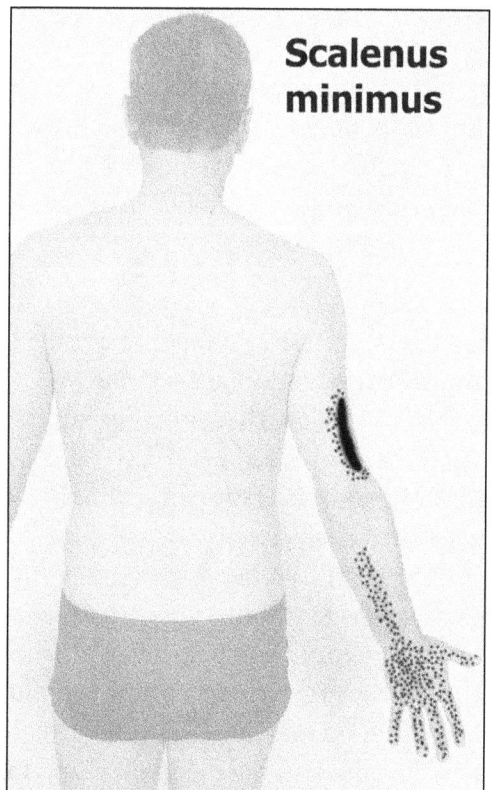
Back referral pattern

Causes and Perpetuation of Trigger Points

- improper arm rest height
- pulling or lifting, especially with your hands at waist level
- horse-handling or riding
- playing tug-of-war
- hauling ropes while sailing
- competitive swimming
- carrying awkwardly large objects
- playing some musical instruments
- sleeping with your head and neck lower than the rest of your body, as when the bed is tilted
- trigger points in the *levator scapula* or *sternocleidomastoid* (chapter 8) muscles
- whiplash from a car accident, or falling on your head
- limping
- improper breathing techniques
- coughing due to an acute or chronic illness
- pain from a bulging or herniated cervical disc, which may linger even after surgery
- a shorter leg or small hemipelvis (either the left or right half of the pelvic bone)
- spinal scoliosis (the spine isn't straight)
- an extra rib at the top (a "cervical rib")
- loss of an arm
- surgical removal of a heavy breast

This is a list of perpetuating factors specific only to trigger points in <u>these</u> muscles. For a full list of perpetuating factors that can cause and perpetuate trigger points anywhere in the body and which also apply to these muscles, please see "Appendix A" (found at the end of this book), since some may need to be addressed for lasting pain relief.

Helpful Hints

- Elevate the head of your bed 2 - 3 inches to provide mild traction at night. Multiple pillows will not provide the same effect, and will probably cause more pain. You should get a good non-springy pillow that provides support for the cervical spine and keeps the spine in alignment. A chiropractor's office usually will carry well-designed pillows. Apply heat to the front of your neck before bedtime.
- When getting up from a lying position, roll onto your side first, and when rolling over in bed keep your head on the pillow rather than lifting it.
- Avoid carrying packages in front of your body, or pulling hard on anything.
- Keep cold drafts off of your neck by using a scarf or neck gaiter.
- Make sure your elbow is resting on something, and that you are sitting straight rather than tilted to the side, no matter what your activity.
- When seated, make sure you have good lighting from behind when you read, so your head isn't turned to the side. Don't read in bed.
- If you have difficulty hearing and tend to turn to one side to hear better, turn your entire body to the side, or get a hearing aid if possible.

- Use a headset for the phone, rather than holding it to your ear or cradling it between your ear and shoulder.
- When using a computer, make sure the monitor is straight ahead and at eye level, and your chair arm rests are at the proper height (your elbows and forearms should rest comfortably on the armrests, neither too short so that you lean to one side, nor too tall so that they hike up your shoulders).
- Learn to breathe properly – see the exercise below.
- Eliminate the causes of coughing by treating the underlying illness as quickly as possible (see Perpetuating Factors, Appendix A)
- If you have an anatomically short leg or small hemipelvis (even as little as 3/8" or less), you will need to get fitted by a specialist for lifts to compensate, or it is unlikely you will be able to resolve *scalene* trigger points.
- Even if you have an extra "cervical" rib, relieving the *scalene* trigger points may be enough to eliminate symptoms.

Self-Help Techniques

Applying Pressure

I don't teach self-help pressure to this muscle due to all the major nerves and arteries in the front of the neck. You will need to go to a trained practitioner such as a physical therapist or a massage therapist.

Stretches

If you are doing the *pectoralis* stretch (chapter 5), only do the top two positions and not the bottom one until the *scalene* muscles have improved. If you have an extra cervical rib, only do the top position.

Side-Bending Neck Stretch: You may wish to apply heat prior to this stretch. Lie face-up, with the hand of the side you are stretching pinned under your butt.

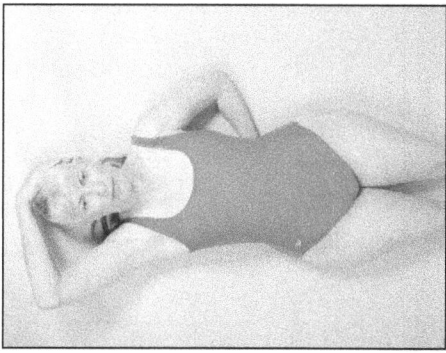

Put your opposite hand over the top of your head and, looking straight at the ceiling, pull your head gently toward your shoulder, then release and take a deep breath.

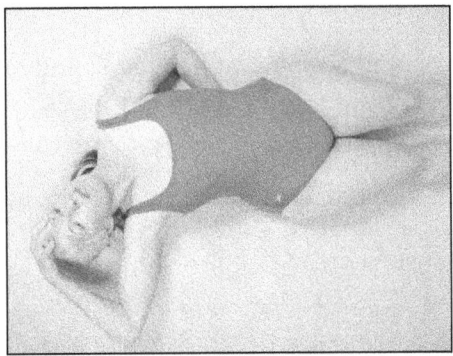

Repeat with your head turned slightly toward the left, and again with your head turned slightly toward the right. This will stretch different parts of the muscle.

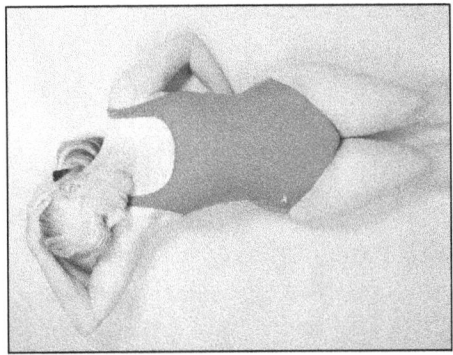 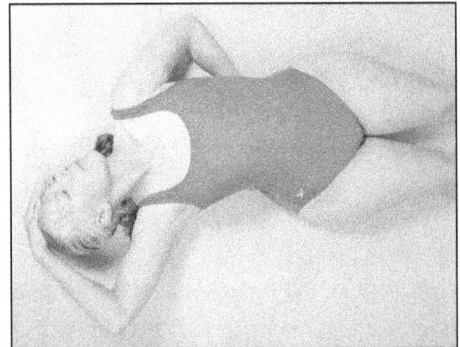

Stretch the opposite side following the same sequence. You may repeat the stretches for each side a few more times.

Scalene Stretch: While sitting up, rotate your head all the way to one side and then bring your chin down. Return to the forward position and take a deep breath. Repeat on the opposite side. You may do this up to four times in each direction.

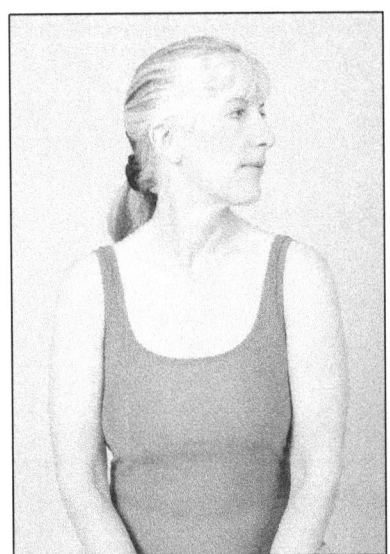 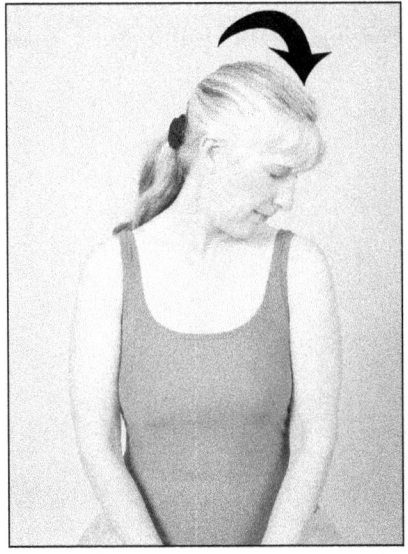

Proper Breathing Exercise: Learning to breathe properly is important for resolving trigger points in several muscles.

Place one hand on your chest and the other on your belly. When you inhale, both hands should rise. As you exhale, both hands should fall. You need to train yourself to notice when you're breathing only into your chest and make sure you start breathing into your belly.

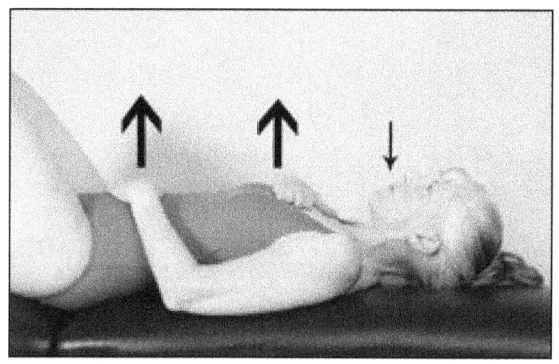 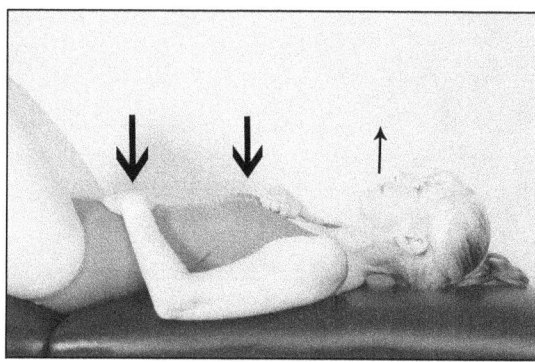

Also See:
* Pectoralis major / subclavius (chapter 5)
* Pectoralis minor (chapter 6)
* Sternocleidomastoid (chapter 8)

You may also need to check the *levator scapula, trapezius, triceps, latissimus dorsi, teres major, subscapularis, deltoid, splenius capitis, brachialis,* hand extensors (*extensors carpi radialis, extensor carpi ulnaris, and extensor digitorum*) and *brachioradialis,* since trigger points in those muscles can either cause similar pain referral patterns or may affect or be affected by *scalene* trigger points in some way. The *splenius capitis* (posterior neck) pressure and stretches can be found in chapter 3.

Since trigger points in these muscles don't directly cause chest of abdominal pain, they are not addressed in this book. If you can't relieve your pain with the self-help techniques in this book after six to eight weeks, you may wish to consider whether you need to treat trigger points in these additional muscles, or if you still have perpetuating factors to resolve. Go to the end of this book for other books by the author that provide self-treatment techniques of muscles not covered in this book.

Differential Diagnosis: If you are unable to relieve your symptoms with trigger point self-help techniques, you may need to see a health care provider to rule out a C_5 to C_6 nerve root irritation. The pain pattern can be very similar to scalene trigger points, or both may be present. You may need to see a chiropractor or osteopathic physician to be evaluated for T_1, C_4, C_5, and C_6 vertebral misalignments, or for elevation of the first rib.

Copyright © 2024 Valerie DeLaune, LAc

Chapter 10: Intercostals / Diaphragm

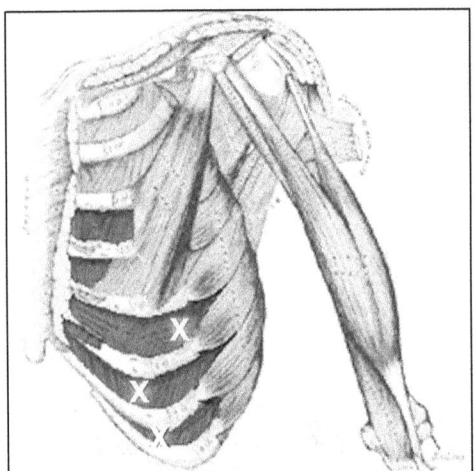
Front view of trunk

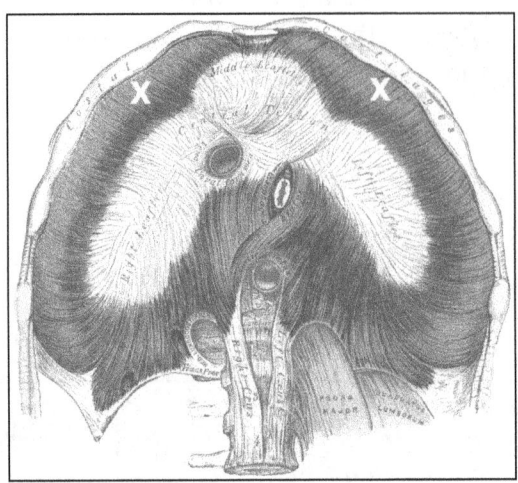
Diaphragm viewed from below in cross-section of trunk, looking up toward lungs

Common Symptoms

Intercostals
- the *intercostal* muscles (in-between each rib) tend to refer aching pain locally and possibly slightly toward the front of your body. More active trigger points may refer pain to the space above and below the adjacent rib.
- you may be unable to lie on the affected side
- pain with attempting to take a deep breath or with full exhalation, and worse with aerobic exercise, coughing, and sneezing
- restricted rotation of the thoracic spine (between the neck and the lumbar area) in one or both directions
- an inability to raise your arm straight up on the affected side due to pain
- pain with bending your trunk away from the side with the trigger points, and pain possibly being partially relieved by bending toward the affected side
- cardiac arrhythmias, including auricular fibrillation, may come from a trigger point in an intercostal muscle on the right side

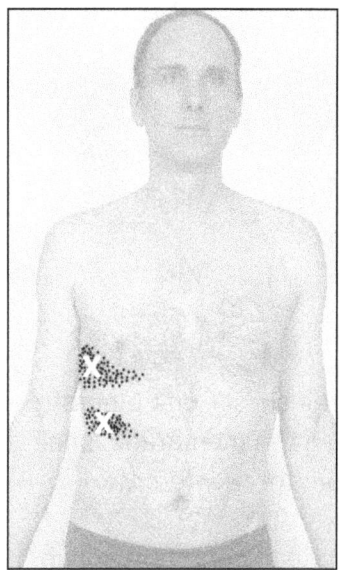
These are examples, but can be found at any level and anywhere around the trunk

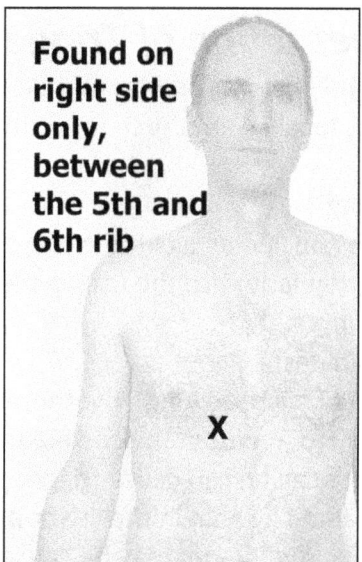
Trigger points can cause cardiac arrhythmias

Diaphragm

- the *diaphragm* (the muscle that forms a wall between the abdominal and thoracic cavities and is used for breathing) causes a "stitch-in-the-side" under the lower border of the rib cage during vigorous exercise, most intense at the end of a full exhalation
- chest pain, difficulty breathing, and an inability to get a full breath, possibly accompanied by a fear of dying if your breathing is severely impaired
- pain with coughing
- pain aggravated by emotional distress
- trigger points in the center of the diaphragm can refer pain to the top of the shoulder on the same side

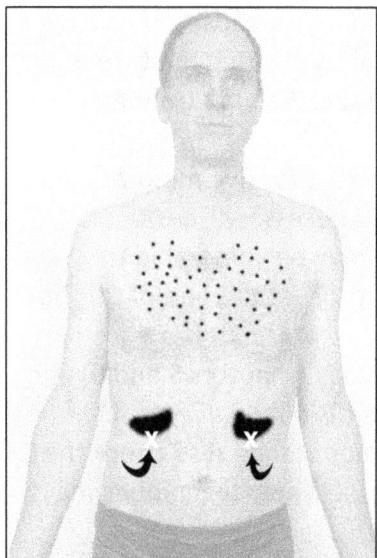
Trigger points are under the edge of the ribcage

Causes and Perpetuation of Trigger Points
- trigger points in the *pectoralis major* muscle (chapter 5)
- trauma, especially local trauma such as an impact
- a broken rib
- improper breathing
- excessive coughing, including a chronic cough
- chest surgery, particularly with the use of chest retractors
- possibly a breast implant
- herpes zoster (shingles)
- a pneumothorax (a collapsed lung), pyothorax (an infection in the chest), or a pleural effusion secondary to a tumor (an accumulation of fluid between the membrane lining the lungs and chest cavity) can cause trigger points in the bottom three *intercostal* muscles, accompanied by pain in the lower part of the chest
- trigger points in the *diaphragm* may be caused by aerobic exercise, a persistent cough, and possibly a gastrectomy (removal of part or all of the stomach)

This is a list of perpetuating factors specific only to trigger points in <u>these</u> muscles. For a full list of perpetuating factors that can cause and perpetuate trigger points anywhere in the body and which also apply to these muscles, please see "Appendix A" (found at the end of this book), since some may need to be addressed for lasting pain relief.

Helpful Hints
- Restoration of proper posture, especially head positioning, is critical to treating trigger points since head-forward posture can both cause and perpetuate trigger points. Head-forward posture can be aggravated while sitting in a car, at a desk, in front of a computer, or while eating dinner or watching TV. Using a good lumbar support everywhere you sit will help correct poor sitting posture. Orthotic inserts in your shoes may improve your standing posture. See chapter 3 for postural re-training.
- If you have a chronic cough, you will need to address the underlying causes. If you are unable to eliminate the cough, you will need to expel phlegm by clearing the throat, or using a cough suppressant. Acupuncture and herbs are very successful at treating coughs and phlegm. See "Appendix A."
- If you must wear some kind of brace around the torso, remove it for five minutes every three hours if possible. Don't wear the brace any longer than necessary.
- If you have been avoiding raising your arm due to pain, you may be vulnerable to developing a "frozen shoulder" (see "Other Books by the Author" at the end of this book for information on this condition).
- Over-doing sit-ups or heavy resistive exercises for the *pectoralis* (chapters 5 and 6) and *biceps* muscles overloads and causes trigger points in the *rectus abdominis* muscle (chapter 11), and may lead to satellite trigger points in the *diaphragm*. Also check the other abdominal muscles (chapter 11) for trigger points; the self-help techniques may help relieve breathing difficulties.

- Trigger points may form in the *intercostal* muscles as a result of an attack of herpes zoster (shingles), and relief of trigger points may be a key factor in relieving post-herpetic pain that is localized, most likely in the rear-outside of the chest.

Self-Help Techniques

Pain while taking a deep breath with the abdomen expanded is more likely to be caused by trigger points in the *transversus abdominis* muscle (chapter 11); pain upon full exhalation with the abdomen pulled in is more likely to be caused by trigger points in the *diaphragm*.

Applying Pressure

Intercostals Pressure: To apply pressure to the intercostal muscles, buy pencil erasers that fit on the end of a pencil. Using the tip of the eraser, press in between the ribs. Hold the pencil in one hand and use the opposite index finger to help you follow the curve of the space in between the ribs.

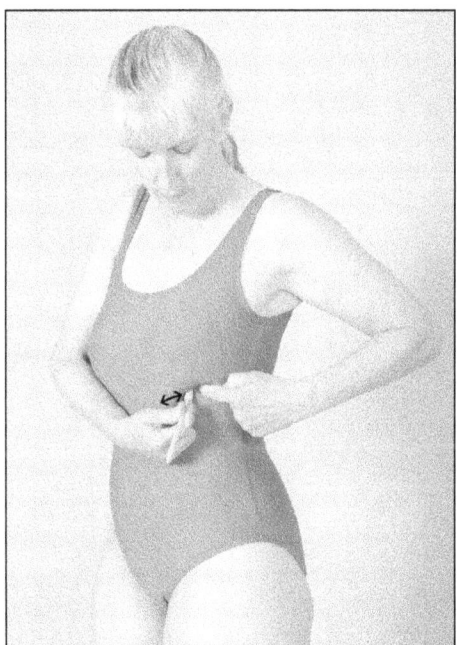

Diaphragm Pressure: To work on the edge of your diaphragm, lie face-up, with your knees bent. Hook the fingers from both hands under the edge of one side of your rib cage, and as you exhale fully, press in and up under your rib cage and pull your ribs outward. Relax and breathe.

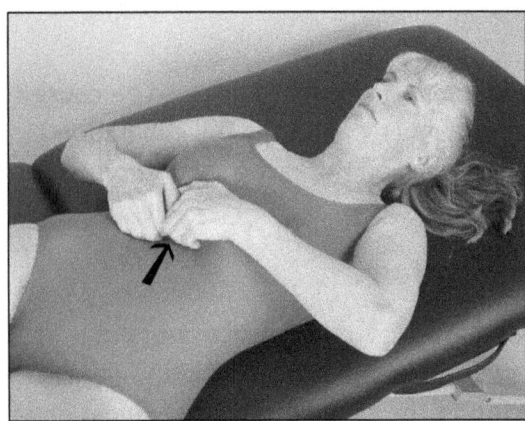

Stretches

Triceps Stretch: To stretch the intercostals, do the triceps stretch and focus on feeling the stretch in the rib cage area. Standing sideways to the wall, place your elbow on the wall above your head, with your forearm bent and your hand behind your head. Lean slightly into the wall to get a gentle stretch.

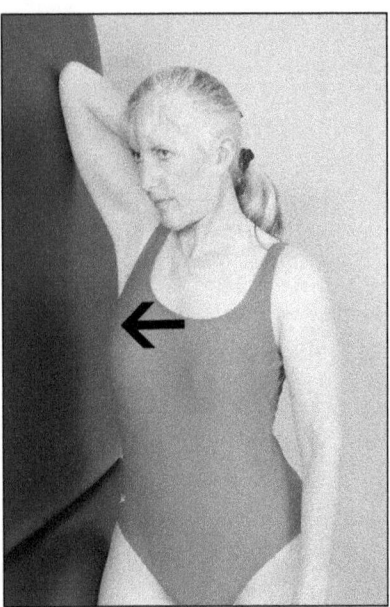

Diaphragm Stretch: To stretch the *diaphragm*, exhale fully and focus on pushing your belly button out. Inhale fully and focus on sucking in the area just below your rib cage. Don't hold these positions—just do the range of motion rhythmically a couple of times.

Copyright © 2024 Valerie DeLaune, LAc

Exercises

Proper Breathing Exercise: Learning to breathe properly is important for resolving trigger points in several muscles; see chapter 9.

Also See:
*   Abdominal muscles (chapter 11)

You may need to check the *serratus anterior* for trigger points after treating the *intercostal* and *diaphragm* muscles. Since trigger points in this muscle don't directly cause chest or abdominal pain, it is not addressed in this book. If you can't relieve your pain with the self-help techniques in this book after six to eight weeks, you may wish to consider whether you need to treat trigger points in this additional muscle, or if you still have perpetuating factors to resolve. Go to the end of this book for other books by the author that provide self-treatment techniques of muscles not covered in this book.

> **Differential Diagnosis:** For conditions that mimic pain from *intercostal* trigger points, or that may be found concurrently, you may need to see a health care provider to rule out heart disease or a heart attack, Tietze's syndrome, thoracic vertebral nerve root irritation, costochondritis, a tumor, pleural effusion, or pyothorax. You may need to see a chiropractor or osteopathic physician to be evaluated for ribs or thoracic vertebrae that are out of alignment. Any of these conditions may be found concurrently with trigger points, so even if you get some relief with trigger point therapy, *you may still need to see a health care provider to ensure that you don't also have a more serious condition.*
>
> For conditions that mimic the pain from *diaphragm* trigger points, you may need to see a health care provider to rule out a diaphragmatic spasm, a peptic ulcer, gastroesophageal reflux, or gallbladder disease if pain is on the right side only.

Chapter 11: Abdominals

(External Abdominal Oblique, Transversus Abdominis, Rectus Abdominis, Pyramidalis)

Trigger points in *abdominal* muscles can cause symptoms such as projectile vomiting, loss of appetite, food intolerance, nausea, belching or burping, heartburn, pain in the bowels, diarrhea, urinary bladder spasms, testicular pain, and painful menses. These symptoms can often be confused with organ problems, but trigger points can be initiated by organ diseases and outlast the disease. You need to rule out organ diseases, and any found need to be treated for lasting relief.

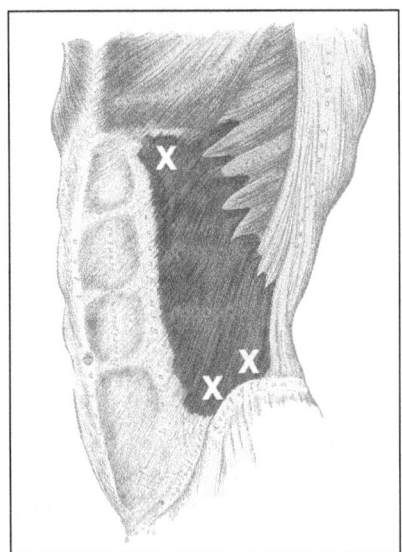
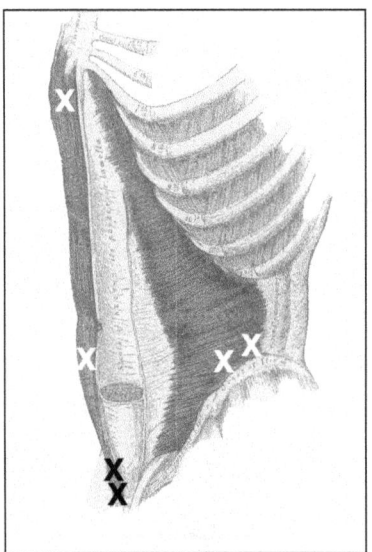

Common Symptoms

- See the pictures for all the referral patterns. These pictures show common trigger points and referral patterns, but trigger points can refer pain or discomfort to the opposite side of the abdomen and even to the back.
- pain that feels like it is in an organ
- often symptoms are described as burning, fullness, bloating, swelling, or excessive gas
- forceful breathing may increase pain

Abdominal Obliques and Transversus Abdominis
- the upper trigger points may produce stomach area pain and/or heartburn and other symptoms commonly associated with a hiatal hernia, but pain is more likely to be continuous, rather than related to the timing of eating or bowel movements
- the lower points may produce urinary frequency, retention of urine, bed-wetting, chronic diarrhea, and groin and testicular pain

- frequent belching and gas, or projectile vomiting (the trigger point is likely found on the back, at or near the bottom of the rib cage)
- restricted trunk rotation

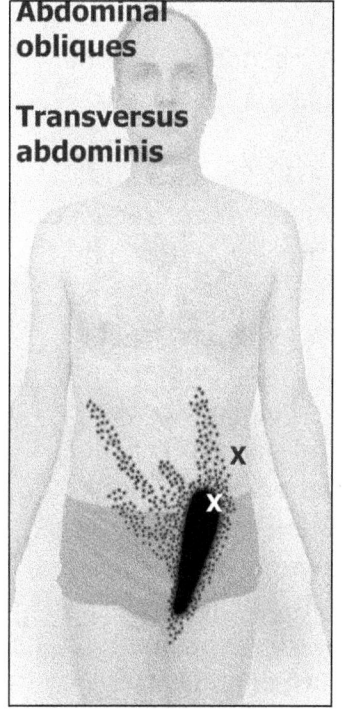

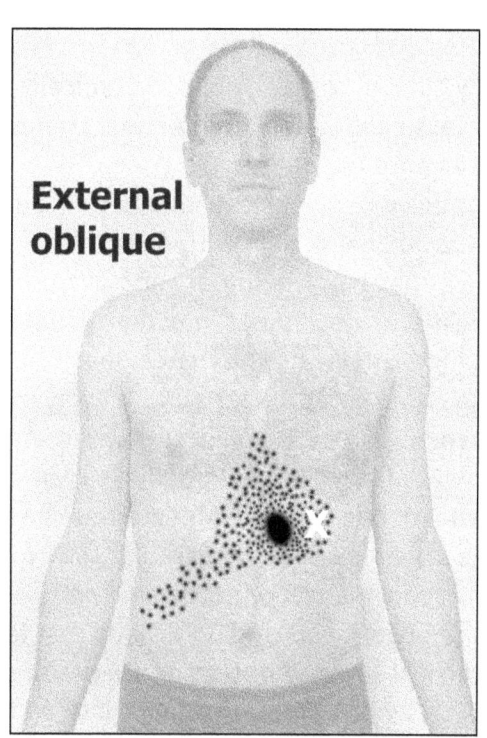

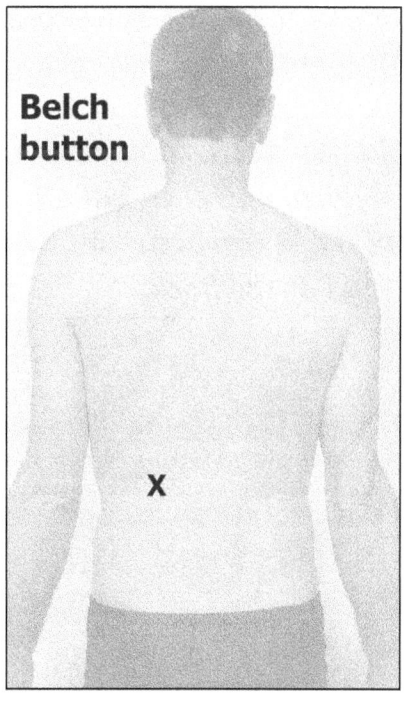

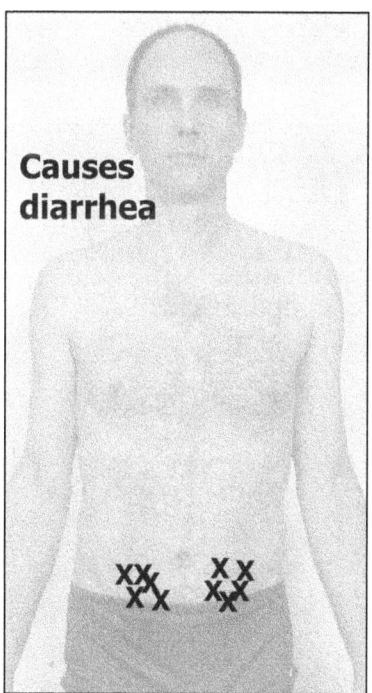

Rectus Abdominis & Pyramidalis
- in the upper portion, symptoms may include referred pain to the mid-back that crosses the back in a horizontal band, abdominal fullness, heartburn, indigestion, heart-area pain, gallbladder-area pain, peptic ulcer-like pain, gynecological-like pain, and sometimes nausea and vomiting
- around the belly button, trigger points are typically aggravated by bending over when lifting, and can cause abdominal or intestinal cramping (if your baby is colicky, try pressing points around the belly button)
- the lower 1/3 of this muscle can cause referred pain that crosses the low back and sacrum in a horizontal band, pain with menses, penis pain, diarrhea, urinary frequency, urinary retention, spasm of the urinary and detrusor sphincter muscles, and pain that *mimics* diverticulitis, kidney stones, and menstrual problems
- "McBurney's" point, usually on the right side a little way down from the level of the belly button and about three-finger's width away from the midline, can cause symptoms that mimic appendicitis. Pain often occurs when the patient is fatigued or worried, or pre-menstrually. At least 12.4% of appendixes removed are normal, and surgery does not solve the pain. In this case, pain is likely due instead to trigger points. However, since a ruptured appendix is life-threatening, you may not have time to rule out trigger points. *With any sudden onset of abdominal pain, go to the emergency room immediately for evaluation*, including a blood test for infection. If you end up having surgery and it did not solve all or part of the problem, search for trigger points.
- "*Rectus Abdominis* syndrome" is entrapment of an anterior branch of a spinal nerve, causing lower abdominal and pelvic pain that simulates gynecological problems in women
- The pyramidalis causes referred pain close to the midline, between the belly button and the top of the pubic bone

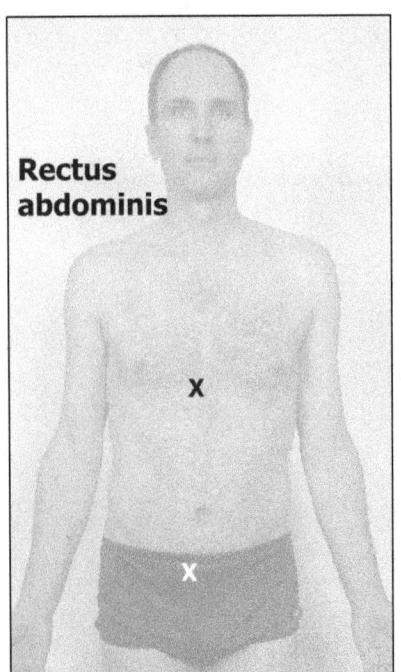

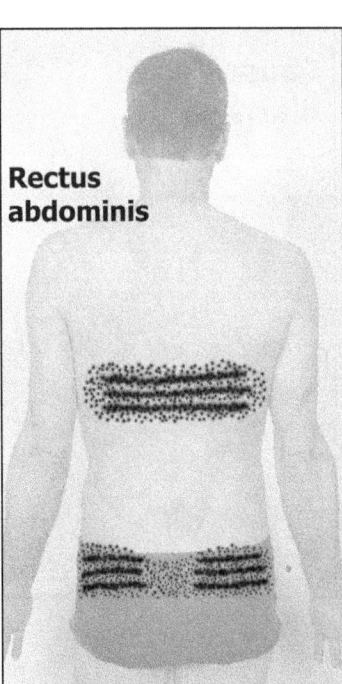

Sample Trigger Points   *Sample Referral Patterns*

Sample rectus abdominis referral patterns, but all of these can occur at any level of the back.

Copyright © 2024 Valerie DeLaune, LAc

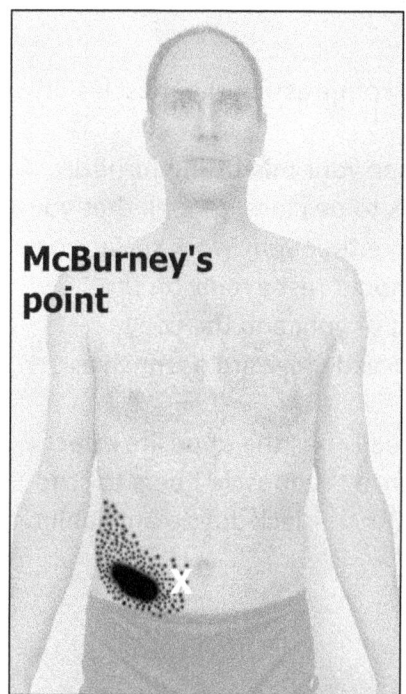
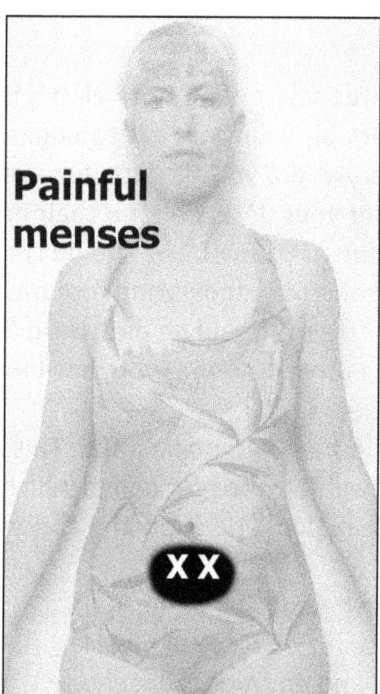
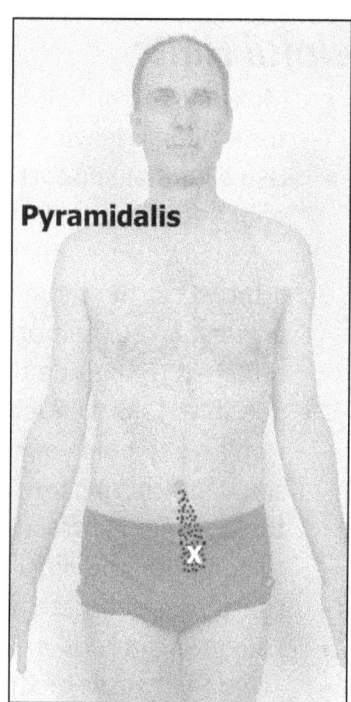

Causes and Perpetuation of Trigger Points

- poor posture such as bending over for long periods of time, your back not being supported, or rotating to one side to see your computer screen
- improper conditioning (i.e., too many sit-ups too soon)
- trying to hold your abdomen in continuously
- a tight belt
- emotional stress
- overall fatigue
- straining due to constipation
- exposure to cold temperatures (due to tensing up)
- direct trauma to the abdominal area, including surgeries such as appendectomies or hysterectomies
- viral infections
- trigger points can be initiated by organ diseases such as a peptic ulcer, intestinal parasites (such as *Entamoeba histolytica*, and beef or fish tapeworms), dysentery (diarrhea caused most likely by drinking unclean water), diverticulosis, diverticulitis, and gallstones, and trigger points may cause symptoms that outlast the organ disease even after resolution of the disease
- a short leg or small hemipelvis (either the right or left half of the pelvis)

This is a list of perpetuating factors specific only to trigger points in these muscles. For a full list of perpetuating factors that can cause and perpetuate trigger points anywhere in the body and which also apply to these muscles, please see "Appendix A" (found at the end of this book), since some may need to be addressed for lasting pain relief.

Helpful Hints

- Make sure your belt, waistband, or pantyhose elastic isn't compressing the muscles. If something is leaving a mark on your skin, it is too tight.
- Use a lumbar support everywhere you sit. Modify or replace your mis-fitting furniture. Your knees should fit under your desk, and the chair needs to be close enough that you can lean against your backrest. Your elbows should rest on either your work surface or armrests at the same height. Your elbows and forearms should rest evenly on the armrests. Your computer screen should be directly in front of you, and the copy attached to the side of the screen, so that you may look directly forward as much as possible. Take frequent breaks.
- Don't try to hold your abdomen in to make it flat. This actually has the opposite effect, since the chronic tension will form trigger points which cause the muscle fibers to stop their proper contraction function, and allow the abdomen to go slack due to an inability to condition the muscles.
- Learn proper breathing techniques (chapter 9).
- Laughter is a good exercise for *abdominal* muscles.
- Treat the causes of stress and emotional upsets.
- Too many sit-ups can not only cause trigger points in the *abdominal* muscles, but can lead to satellite trigger points in the *diaphragm* muscle as well (the muscle that divides the thoracic cavity and the abdominal cavity, chapter 10)
- Learn proper conditioning techniques, either with the help of a physical therapist or other trained specialist who knows how to modify an activity for your set of circumstances. Don't overdo conditioning exercises. You shouldn't do activities that are painful, or make you sore later. It is better to add repetitions and increase weights *slowly* so that you make steady progress, rather than hurt yourself and have to stop until you are well again.
- Treat the cause of constipation. Acupuncture and herbs are very successful at treating constipation.
- Head-forward posture can be a result of trigger points in the *upper rectus abdominis* muscle.
- Treat organ diseases such as ulcers, gallstones, parasites, and diverticulitis.
- Scars left from surgeries usually cause numerous trigger points in the surrounding muscles, so check for trigger points around any abdominal scars. Acupuncture scar treatments are very effective for treating these trigger points, even years after the surgery.

Self-Help Techniques

Abdominal pain may be trigger point referral from the *paraspinal* muscles (chapter 3), and pain in the back may be referred from trigger points in the *abdominal* muscles, so you should check both sets of muscles. Gastrointestinal pain and cramping, and nausea and belching may also be due to trigger points in the *paraspinal* muscles (chapter 3). Lower abdominal pain, tenderness, and muscle spasming may also come from trigger points located in the vaginal wall (see *pelvic floor* muscles, chapter 13).

Applying Pressure

Abdominal Pressure: Lying face-up, use your fingers to apply pressure to sensitive points in the entire abdominal area. You may find it easier if you have a pillow under your knees. Be sure to check all the way from the bottom rib to the top of the pubic bone, and out to the sides. When working on the top edge of the pubic bone, press down toward your feet rather than toward your back. You may combine this with applying hot packs or sitting in a warm bath.

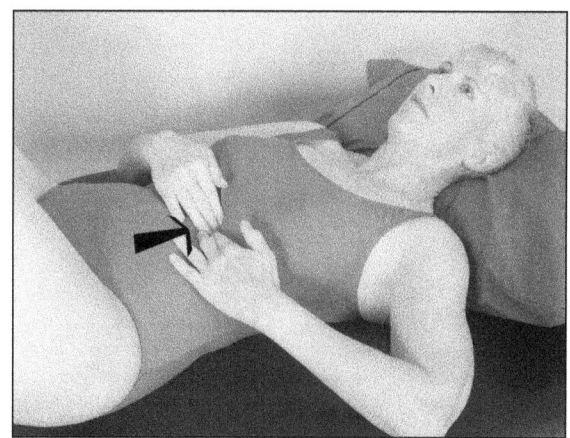

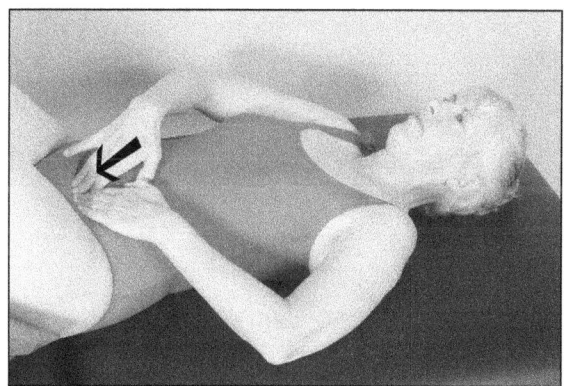

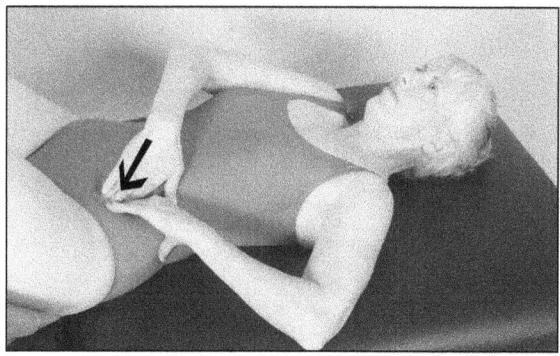

Stretches

Abdominal Stretch: Use something round such as a large inflatable therapeutic exercise ball (from a chiropractor or physical therapist) or a concrete form tube (from a building supply store). Lie face-up over it with your arms outstretched over your head and touch your palms to the floor. Be careful not to fall over, and don't do this stretch if you are elderly or pregnant. I find the concrete form tube easier to use, since you can't roll off to the side. You may not be able to perform this stretch if you have back problems.

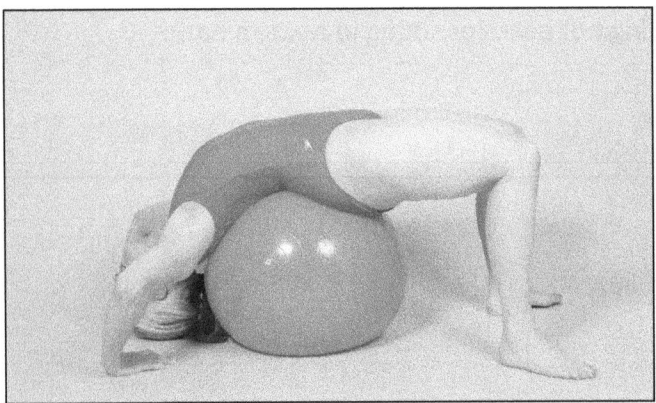

Hip-Extension Stretch: As an alternative to the Abdominal Stretch, lie face-down on a flat surface, such as the floor. Using your arms, push your torso off of the surface with your head looking straight ahead at the wall, but keep your pelvis on the surface. If you can only rest on your elbows, you will still get a stretch. Breathe deeply to expand your abdomen. You may not be able to do this stretch if you have neck or shoulder girdle problems.

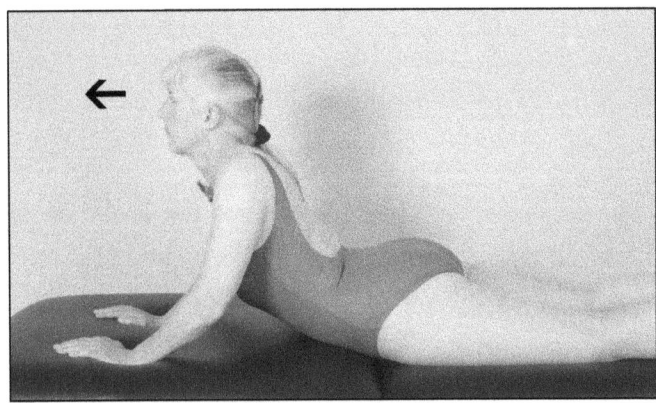

Exercises

Pelvic Tilt Exercise: The pelvic tilt strengthens the *rectus abdominis*. Once trigger points have been inactivated for a few weeks, you may add this conditioning exercise. With this exercise, be sure to rest between each repetition for an equal amount of time it took to perform the repetition.

Lie face-up with your knees bent, with one hand over your lower abdomen and one hand above your navel.

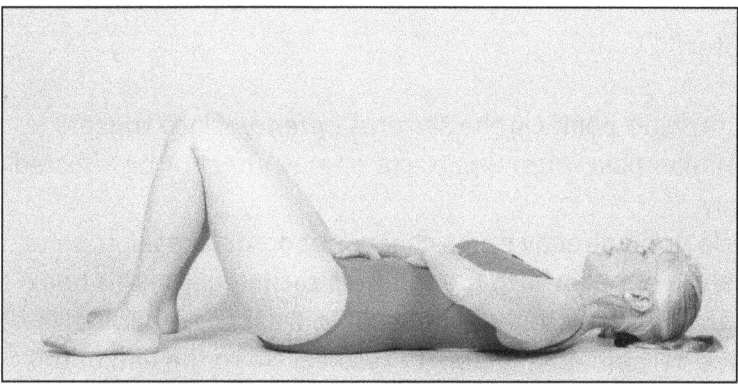

First flatten out the lumbar area of your back against the floor, which brings the two hands closer together.

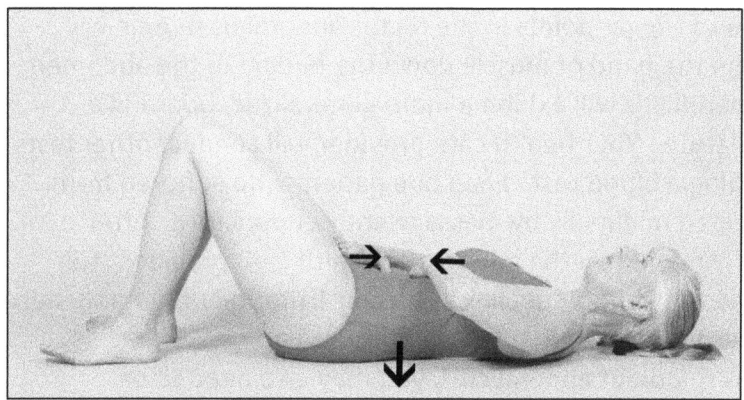

Then push your butt off the floor so only your feet and mid to upper back are still on the floor—the hands should come even closer together. If your hands get further apart, you are arching your back rather than flattening it correctly.

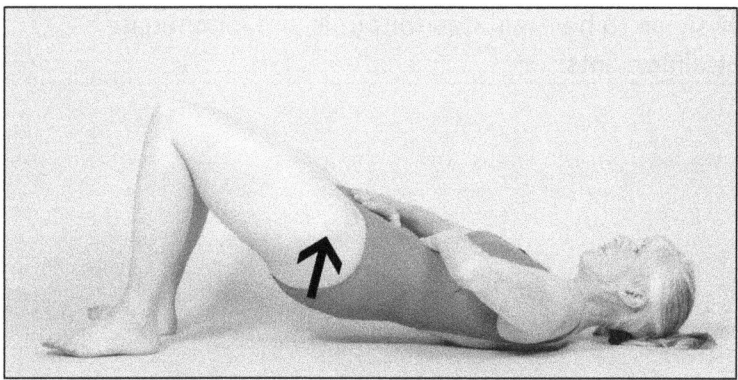

Finally, roll back down to relax on the floor and take a deep breath.

Also See:
* Paraspinal (chapter 3)
* Diaphragm (chapter 11)
* Adductor Muscles of the Hip (chapter 12)

You may also need to search for trigger points in the *serratus anterior*, since trigger points in this muscle can either cause similar pain referral patterns or may affect or be affected by *abdominal* trigger points in some way.

Since trigger points in this muscle don't directly cause chest or abdominal pain, it is not addressed in this book. If you can't relieve your pain with the self-help techniques in this book after six to eight weeks, you may wish to consider whether you need to treat trigger points in this additional muscle, or if you still have perpetuating factors to resolve. Go to the end of this book for other books by the author that provide self-treatment techniques of muscles not covered in this book.

> **Differential Diagnosis:** *If you are experiencing sudden abdominal pain, go to the emergency room!* Abdominal pain more likely due to trigger points in the rectus abdominis muscle will exhibit palpable nodules and ropiness in the band of muscle down the middle of the abdomen. Abdominal pain more likely due to appendicitis will exhibit a more generalized, board-like rigidity in the entire abdominal musculature. Your health care provider will conduct other tests to evaluate you for appendicitis, including a blood test. I had one patient who suffered from low-grade abdominal pain that was helped minimally by massage and acupuncture. After several months, she had her appendix removed on the advice of a health care provider. Her pain was relieved, and it was determined she had a subclinical chronic irritation of her appendix with fibrous tissues, even though it was not diseased.
>
> Once a health care provider has ruled out appendicitis, you may also need to be evaluated for a peptic ulcer, colitis, painful rib syndrome, urinary tract disease, fibromyalgia, a hiatal hernia, gastric carcinoma, kidney or gallstones, an inguinal hernia, hepatitis, pancreatitis, gynecological disorders, diverticulosis, an umbilical hernia, thoracic or upper lumbar nerve root irritation, costochondritis, ascariasis, epilepsy, and rectus abdominis hematoma. Pain in the upper abdomen may be caused by Tietze's syndrome or slipping rib syndrome. You may need to see a chiropractor or osteopathic physician to be evaluated for pubic and innominate dysfunctions or for vertebral and rib misalignments.

Chapter 12: Adductor Muscles of the Hip

*(Adductor Longus, Adductor Brevis,
Adductor Magnus, and Gracilis)*

This chapter is in included in this book because *adductor magnus* trigger points can refer to the inside the pelvis (see below).

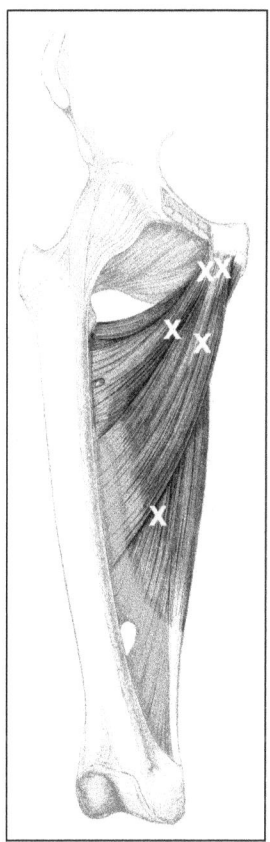

*Front view of thigh --
Adductor muscles*

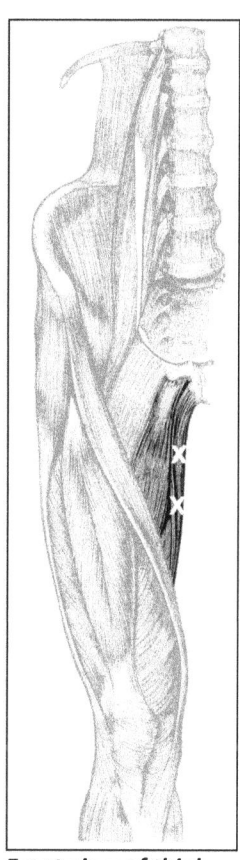

*Front view of thigh --
Gracilis*

Common Symptoms

Adductor Longus and Adductor Brevis
- referred pain on the front of your thigh, over the front of your knee, and down the inside of your lower leg
- pain feels deep
- trigger points may cause stiffness of your knee
- possibly pain may only be felt during vigorous activity or muscle overload
- pain is increased by standing and by sudden twists of your hip
- restricted range-of-motion in moving your thigh away from the midline of your body
- possibly restricted range-of-motion in rotating your thigh outward

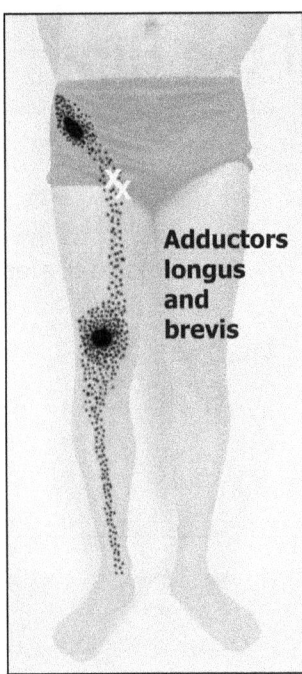

Adductors longus and brevis

Adductor Magnus
- pain on the front-inside of your thigh, from your groin area down to the inside of your knee
- pain feels deep, possibly like it's shooting up into your pelvis and exploding like a firecracker
- the common trigger point high up between the legs may refer pain to your pubic bone, vagina, rectum, or possibly your bladder
- pain may only occur during intercourse
- difficulty getting comfortable at night

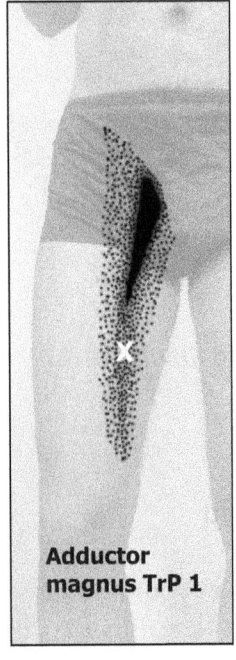

Adductor magnus TrP 1

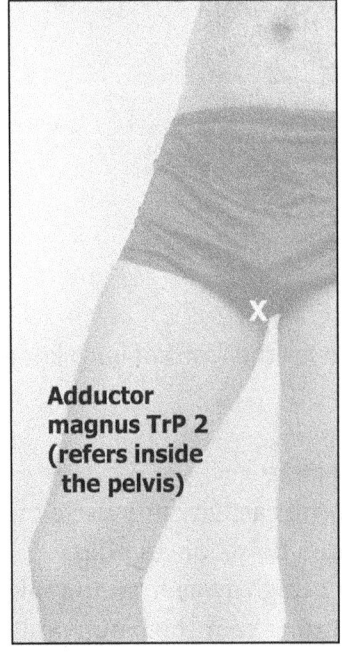

Adductor magnus TrP 2 (refers inside the pelvis)

Gracilis
- pain on the inside of your thigh that feels hot, stingy, and superficial
- pain may be constant at rest, and no change of position relieves it except for walking

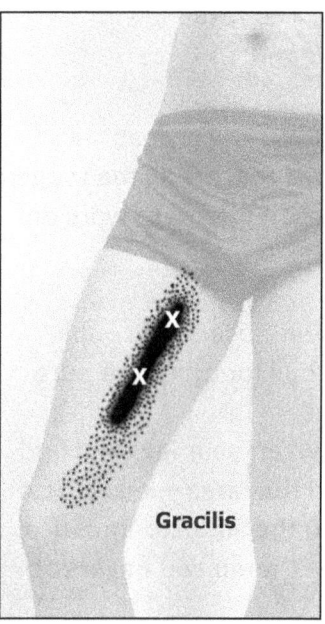

Causes and Perpetuation of Trigger Points
- a sudden overload, for example, trying to stop yourself from slipping on ice by trying to keep your legs from spreading
- horseback riding
- long bike trips (if you haven't trained for it)
- running up or down hills
- sitting for long periods, especially when driving, or with one leg crossed over the other knee
- skiing (most likely by snowplowing/wedge turns, or unexpectedly doing the "splits")

This is a list of perpetuating factors specific only to trigger points in <u>these</u> muscles. For a full list of perpetuating factors that can cause and perpetuate trigger points anywhere in the body and which also apply to these muscles, please see "Appendix A" (found at the end of this book), since some may need to be addressed for lasting pain relief.

Helpful Hints
- Be sure to read the section on perpetuating factors in Appendix A, particularly the sections on infections, nutritional problems, and organ dysfunction and disease.
- When sleeping, put a pillow between your knees, and try to keep your upper leg almost straight.
- Don't sit with your legs crossed, and if you must sit for long periods, stand and move around frequently.

Self-Help Techniques

Apply moist heat to the upper front and inner thigh.

Applying Pressure

Parts of these muscles are more difficult to treat on yourself, so you will probably also need the help of a massage therapist, acupuncturist, or physical therapist to treat all the trigger points. Since the *adductors magnus* and *brevis* trigger points are so deep, it is hard to work on these muscles with massage alone. Ultrasound is an effective treatment.

Hip Adductor Pressure: Sit with your legs bent to one side, with one heel close to the pubic area and the other one out to the side. Use your fingers or press a golf ball (or other pressure device in the center of your palm) into tender points on your inner thigh.

To access the upper portion of the adductor magnus, reach between your legs and find your sit bone with your fingers. Press the muscle attachment all around that area—it is easiest to use the hand of the opposite side. In addition to applying pressure to the adductor muscles, you may be able to lift and pinch part of this muscle group between the thumb and fingers of your opposite hand.

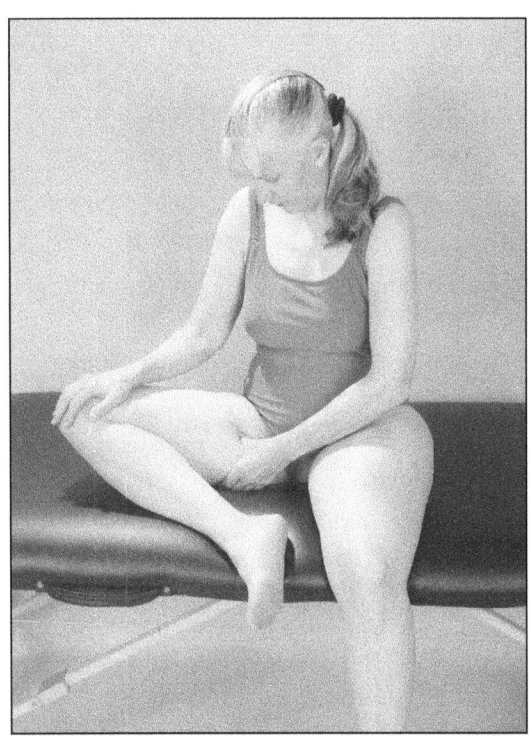

Stretches

Hip Adductor Stretch: Hold onto a chair back, spread your legs apart almost as far as you can with your toes pointed straight forward, and gently rotate your pelvis away from the side you are stretching.

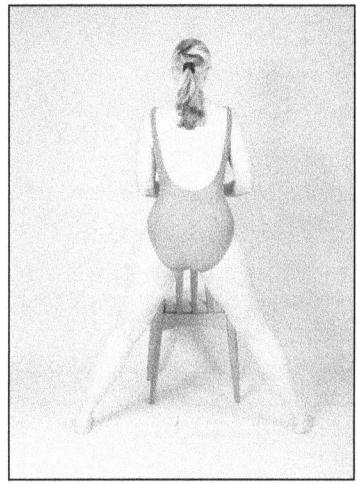 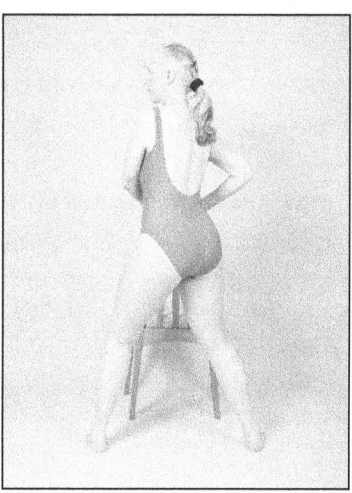 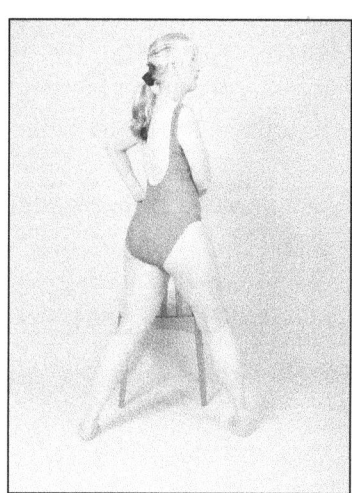

Pool Adductor Stretch: Hold onto a chair back, spread your legs apart almost as far as you can, and shift your weight to one side, allowing that knee to bend. The stretch is felt on the opposite inner thigh. It may be easier on your knees to do this stretch in a warm swimming pool in chest-deep water.

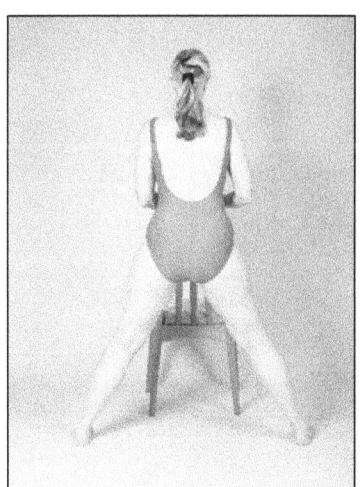 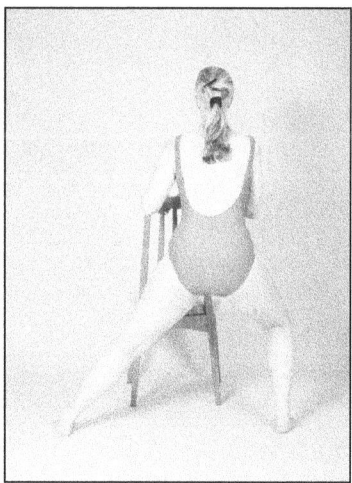 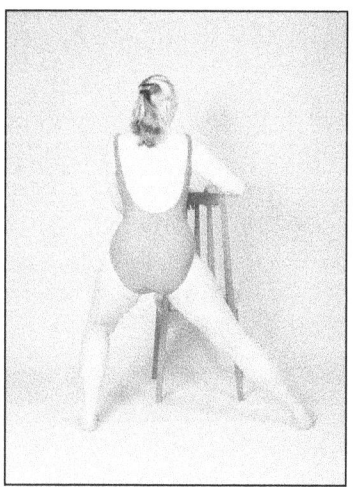

Also See:

You may also need to search for trigger points in the *vastus lateralis*, since trigger points in that muscle can affect or be affected by *hip adductor* trigger points. Since trigger points in this muscle doesn't directly cause chest or abdominal pain, it is not addressed in this book. If you can't relieve your pain with the self-help techniques in this book after six to eight weeks, you may wish to consider whether you need to treat trigger points in this additional muscle, or if you still have perpetuating factors to resolve. Go to the end of this book for other books by the author that provide self-treatment techniques of muscles not covered in this book.

Differential Diagnosis: Three conditions may overload the hip adductors and cause chronic problems: pubic stress symphysitis, pubic stress fracture, and adductor insertion avulsion syndrome. If you are not able to relieve trigger points more than temporarily, you should see a health care provider to check for these conditions.

Also See:

Chapter 13: Pelvic Floor

*(Sphincter Ani, Transverse Perinei, Levator Ani,
Coccygeus, Ischiocavernosus, Bulbospongiosus, Obturator Internus)*

Though there is little you can do for self-help for the *pelvic floor* muscles for application of pressure to trigger points, because the symptoms can be so distressing and so poorly diagnosed in relation to trigger points, I am including a chapter so you can find a professional (most likely a physical therapist trained in intra-pelvic trigger points) that can evaluate the presence of trigger points and their perpetuating factors. Women are far more affected than men -- in a group of 100 patients, 83% will be women.

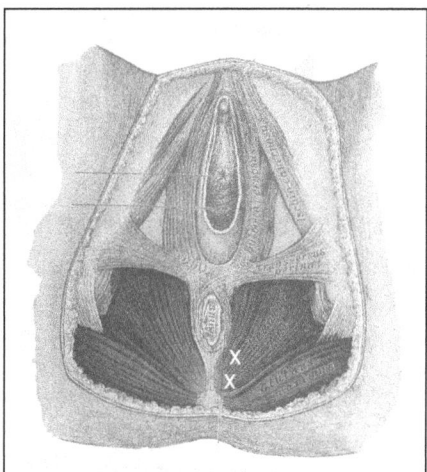 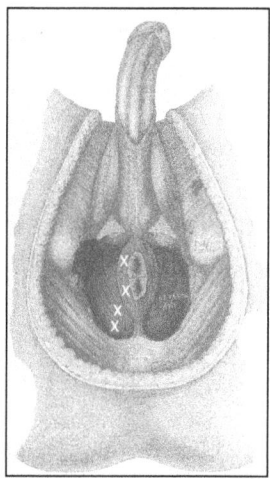 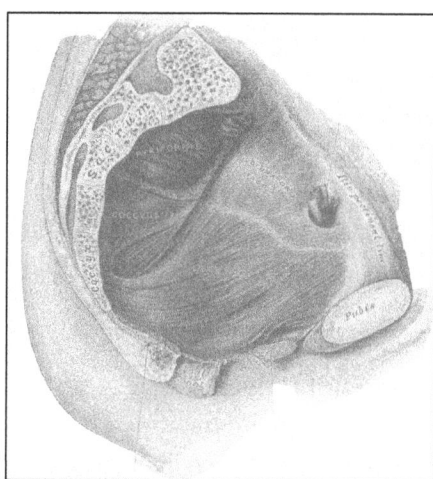

Common Symptoms

Sphincter Ani
- it's hard for the patient to explain exactly where the pain is, and usually describe it as tailbone, hip, or back pain
- the area of referred pain includes the tailbone and often includes the anal area and the lower part of the sacrum (the triangular bone between the lumbar vertebrae and the tailbone)
- possibly painful bowel movements

Transverse Perinei
- it's hard for the patient to explain exactly where the pain is, and usually describe it as tailbone, hip, or back pain
- the area of referred pain includes the tailbone and often includes the anal area and the lower part of the sacrum (the triangular bone between the lumbar vertebrae and the tailbone)

Levator Ani (includes the pubococcygeus and iliococcygeus muscles)
- it's hard for the patient to explain exactly where the pain is, and usually describe it as tailbone, hip, or back pain
- the area of referred pain includes the tailbone and often includes the anal area and the lower part of the sacrum (the triangular bone between the lumbar vertebrae and the tailbone)
- trigger points may cause vaginal pain, especially during intercourse
- trigger points may cause rectal pain or pain inside the pelvis
- sitting may be uncomfortable, and pain may be aggravated by lying on the back and by bowel movements
- there may possibly be a relationship with constipation or frequent bowel movements
- pain may be diagnosed as "coccygodynia," although the tailbone itself is usually normal and not tender
- pain may also be diagnosed as "levator ani syndrome" or other similar terms

Coccygeus
- it's hard for the patient to explain exactly where the pain is, and usually describe it as tailbone, hip, or back pain
- the area of referred pain includes the tailbone and often includes the anal area and the lower part of the sacrum (the triangular bone between the lumbar vertebrae and the tailbone)
- pain may be diagnosed as "coccygodynia," although the tailbone itself is usually normal and not tender
- sitting may be painful
- trigger points are likely to a cause myofascial backache late in pregnancy and early on in labor

Ischiocavernosus
- trigger points are likely to refer pain to the genital area, such as the vagina and the base of the penis beneath the scrotum
- referred pain in the area between the scrotum or vagina and the anus

Bulbospongiosus
- trigger points are likely to refer pain to the genital area, such as the vagina and the base of the penis beneath the scrotum
- in women, possibly pain with intercourse, particularly during entry
- in women, possibly aching pain in the area between the vagina and the anus
- in men, possibly pain in the region of the backside of the scrotum, discomfort sitting erect, and sometimes a degree of impotence

Obturator Internus (intrapelvic portion)
- trigger points may cause vaginal pain
- pain may be referred to the anal and tailbone areas, and to the upper back of the thigh
- there may be referred pain and a feeling of fullness in the rectum

Post-surgical Vaginal Wall Trigger Points
- after a hysterectomy, trigger points may form in the vaginal wall which can refer pain to the lower abdomen and uterine paracervical area
- the patient usually describes the pain in what is familiar terms to them: "ovarian pain," "menstrual cramps," or "bladder spasms," and pressure on the vaginal trigger points reproduces the symptoms

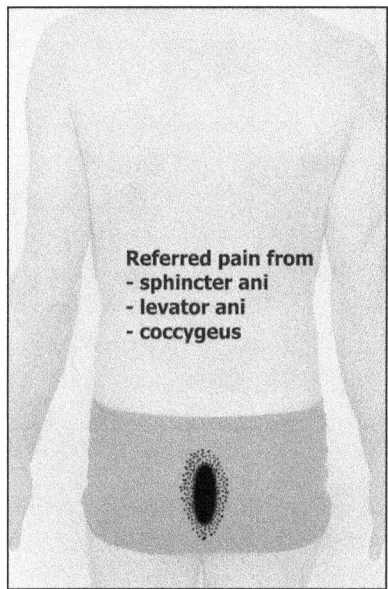
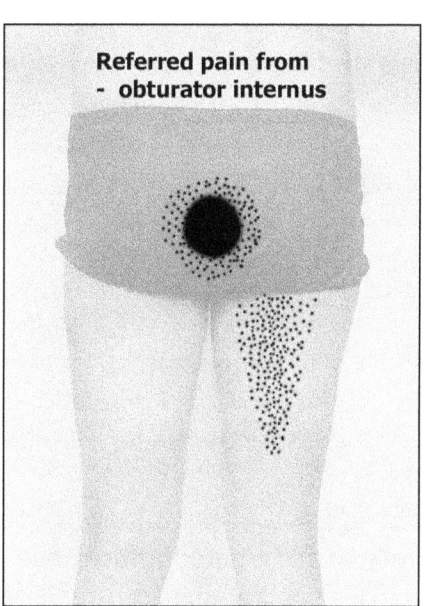

Causes and Perpetuation of Trigger Points
- Muscle spasm and tenderness can be caused by articular dysfunction at the sacroiliac junction (the slightly moveable joint where the sacrum and the big pelvic bone meets isn't moving properly). Also, trigger points in the *pelvic floor* muscles that attach to the sacrum can destabilize the sacroiliac joint.
- Trigger points in the pelvic region can be activated by a severe fall, an auto accident, or surgery in the pelvic region.
- Most of the time it is impossible for the patient to identify a particular event that triggered the pain. In these cases, nutritional or other systemic perpetuating factors need to be identified and addressed; see "Appendix A" at the end of this book.
- *Levator ani* trigger points can be activated by sitting with a slumped posture for long periods.
- Chronic inflammation such as hemorrhoids, endometriosis, chronic salpingo-oophoritis, chronic prostatovesiculitis, and interstitial cystitis have been associated with *levator ani* spasm syndrome.

This is a list of perpetuating factors specific only to trigger points in these muscles. For a full list of perpetuating factors that can cause and perpetuate trigger points anywhere in the body and which also apply to these muscles, please see "Appendix A" (found at the end of this book), since some may need to be addressed for lasting pain relief.

Helpful Hints

- Sit upright with proper lumbar support.
- See a health care provider to identify and treat any chronic inflammations such as hemorrhoids, endometriosis, chronic salpingo-oophoritis, chronic prostatovesiculitis, and interstitial cystitis.
- See a chiropractor or osteopathic physician to identify and treat dysfunctions of the lumbrosacral, sacroiliac, and sacrococcygeal joints.
- Some physical therapists specialize in treating *pelvic* muscles, and use a variety of techniques including strengthening programs.

Treatment Techniques (for Practitioners)

Applying Pressure

The coccygeal region and the *coccygeus* muscle are more difficult to palpate from the vagina than the rectum because of the two layers of rectal mucosa and one layer of vaginal mucosa. For this reason, *a good exam and treatment must include both rectal and vaginal exams.*

The *sphincter ani*, *levator ani*, *coccygeus*, *obturator internus*, and *sacrococcygeus ventralis* muscles are best examined and treated through the rectum. First check for hemorrhoids, since they can make examination painful and be a cause of trigger points. If the anal sphincter has trigger points, this can also cause a great deal of pain, so the solution is to have the patient bear down to enhance relaxation as the practitioner slowly inserts a finger. If this is still too painful, try a vaginal exam.

In women, the *bulbospongiosus* muscle can only be examined vaginally. Parts of the *coccygeus* and *obturator internus* can be better examined vaginally. *The transversus perinei*, *ischiocavernosus*, and *bulbospongiosus* are examined externally in men, and the first two examined externally in women.

A detailed explanation of the examination of *pelvic floor* muscles is found in *Myofascial Pain and Dysfunction: The Trigger Point Manual, Vol. 2, The Lower Extremities* (Travell and Simons 1992, pp. 110–29).

Also See:

You may also need to search for trigger points in the *gluteus maximus* and *piriformis*, since trigger points in those muscles can either cause similar pain referral patterns or may affect or be affected by pelvic floor trigger points in some way.

Since trigger points in these muscles don't directly cause chest or abdominal pain, they are not addressed in this book. If you can't relieve your pain with the self-help techniques in this book after six to eight weeks, you may wish to consider whether you need to treat trigger points in these additional muscles, or if you still have perpetuating factors to resolve. Go to the end of this book for other books by the author that provide self-treatment techniques of muscles not covered in this book.

APPENDIX A

What Causes and Keeps Trigger Points Going: Perpetuating Factors

> "If we treat myofascial pain syndromes without . . . correcting the multiple perpetuating factors, the patient is doomed to endless cycles of treatment and relapse. [Perpetuating factors are] the most neglected part of the management of myofascial pain syndromes . . . The answer to the question, 'How long will the beneficial results of specific myofascial therapy last?', depends largely on what perpetuating factors remain unresolved . . . One may view perpetuating factors also as predisposing factors, since their presence tends to make the muscles more susceptible to the activation of [trigger points] . . . Usually, one stress activates the [trigger point], then other factors perpetuate it. In some patients, these perpetuating factors are so important that their elimination results in complete relief of the pain without any local treatment."   ~~ *Doctors Janet Travell and David G. Simons*

There is much more to "Neuromuscular Therapy" or "Trigger Point Therapy" than learning referral patterns and how to search for trigger points; it is very important for a health care provider to identify and figure out *with* the patient what is causing and perpetuating their symptoms. This requires getting a complete medical history and evaluating for any potential perpetuating factors.

Trigger points are a *symptom*, not a *cause*. Needling or applying pressure to the trigger points treats the acute part of the problem, but does not resolve the underlying factors. If you get temporary relief from trigger point therapy but symptoms quickly recur, then trigger points are definitely a factor, but perpetuating factors need to be addressed in order to gain lasting relief.

This appendix will outline some general causes of trigger point activation and how to address the factors, and each muscle chapter will specifically address issues particularly pertinent to that muscle. I recommend you read all of the perpetuating factors, since you likely have more than one factor that you may not have recognized up to this point.

Acute or Chronic Viral, Bacterial, and Parasitic Infections

Acute infections, such as **colds, flu, strep throat, and bronchitis** will aggravate trigger points, particularly in a person with fibromyalgia or chronic fatigue. It is important to head off illness at the first sign in order to avoid perpetuating trigger points. When you start to get sick, take the Chinese herbs Gan Mao Ling or Yin Chiao, Echinacea, and/or homeopathics such as Osillococcinum or other appropriate homeopathics for colds, flu, or sinusitis. Once you are past the initial stage of illness, if symptoms progress, the Chinese herbs you take will be determined by your particular set of symptoms, so at this point you may need professional help to determine the proper herbs. You should have the above-mentioned herbs and homeopathics available at home so you can treat your symptoms as soon as you notice the first signs. This is particularly important if you have fibromyalgia, sinusitis, asthma, or other recurrent infections, since your trigger points will be activated by illness, and getting sick can set you back by weeks in your treatment and healing.

Outbreaks of **chronic infections**, such as **herpes simplex** (cold sores, genital herpes, herpes zoster) will also aggravate trigger points, and may need to be managed if recurrence is frequent. There are many pharmaceutical drugs and natural supplements/herbs for treating recurrent herpes infections, and some will work better than others for you. Also, if you are getting recurrent outbreaks you will want figure out what is stressing your immune system, such as allergies or emotional stress. Sometimes a herpes outbreak is the first sign you are fighting an acute illness, so that is the time to take the above-mentioned supplements.

Other chronic infections such as **sinus infections, an abscessed or impacted tooth, or urinary tract infections** will perpetuate trigger points. If you suspect a **tooth**, you will need to see your dentist for evaluation. **Urinary tract infections** (UTI's) need to be dealt with promptly. You may use over-the-counter western drugs, Chinese herbs, and cranberry (don't use sweetened juice), but if you don't respond to treatment immediately you will need to see your health care provider, since UTI's can turn into life-threatening kidney infections. Any mechanical reasons for **sinus infections** need to be dealt with for lasting relief. Naturopathic doctors can use a small inflatable balloon to open up the passages. You may need surgical intervention if the blockage is severe enough. Many people report success using a Neti Pot (get it at your health food store) to flush the sinuses with a warm saline solution. With both sinus infections and UTI's, antibiotics often won't kill all of the pathogens, and you may get a lingering, recurrent infection. However, antibiotics also work quickly, so I often recommend to patients that they combine antibiotics, acupuncture, herbs, and homeopathics to knock the infection out as quickly and completely as possible so it doesn't become a chronic problem.

The fish tapeworm, giardia, and occasionally amoeba are the most likely **parasites** to perpetuate trigger points. The fish tapeworm and giardia scar the lining of the intestine and impair your ability to absorb nutrients, and they also consume vitamin B-12. **Amoeba** can produce toxins that are passed from the intestine into the body. **Fish tapeworms** can be transmitted from raw fish. **Giardia** is most often associated with drinking untreated water from streams, but it can also be passed by an infected person not washing their hands after a bowel movement, particularly if they are preparing food or have some other hand-to-mouth contact.

Any time you have **chronic diarrhea** it is worth testing for parasites. A cheaper alternative is just to treat with herbs like grapefruit seed extract or Pulsatilla (a Chinese herb) and see if your symptoms improve. Since these will also kill off the good intestinal flora, you will want to follow treatment with a good multi-acidophilus supplement, as you would after any antibiotic. If you have blood in your stools, you should always see your health care provider immediately to rule out serious conditions. Acupuncture and Naturopathy can help resolve chronic diarrhea from most causes.

There is substantial controversy about whether **systemic candida infections** exist, though it is now listed in the Merck Manual (a medical text of illness and disease). There is abundant information on the Web regarding this subject, so I won't go into detail. Candida is a normal intestinal flora, but can multiply beyond a normal amount and cause a variety of symptoms including muscular pain. Many people report feeling much better on an anti-candida diet, and in any case it is a pretty healthy way to eat. There are many herbal products on the market for eliminating candida, including grapefruit seed extract, oil of oregano, Echinacea, Pulsatilla, and many formulas. Again, you will want to follow any of these with a good multi-acidophilus supplement to replace the beneficial intestinal flora.

Allergies and other Environmental Stressors

Both inhaled and ingested allergens perpetuate trigger points and make them harder to treat due to the subsequent histamine release. Skin tests are useful for testing for **inhaled allergens**, and there are a few methods for testing for **food allergens**.

One of the best ways to test for **food allergens** is an elimination diet, where you eliminate all foods, add them back in one at a time, and then rotate foods. You can find instructions for this in *"Prescription for Nutritional Healing"* by Balch and Balch under "Allergies." The challenge with a rotation diet is that most people are not willing to do it, as it takes a very strict control of your diet and a careful food diary for a month. As an alternative, Balch and Balch offer a quick-test. After sitting and relaxing for a few minutes, take your pulse rate for one minute, then eat the food you are testing. Keep still for 15-20 minutes and take your pulse again. If your pulse rate has increased more than ten beats per minute, eliminate this food from your diet for one month, then re-test. Naturopathic doctors offer a blood test for food sensitivities. Food allergens and sensitivities must be eliminated, but this can become challenging when you eat at other people's homes, when dining out, or while traveling. Try to keep something you *can* have with you, so you have an alternative.

There may be some ingested substances to which you are not allergic, but can aggravate your condition anyway and should be avoided. Chinese diagnosis differentiates pain by the quality of the pain (dull, achy, sharp, shooting, stabbing, burning, moving) and what makes it better or worse (i.e., rest/activity, heat/cold/damp, etc.), and some foods will aggravate certain conditions. You can see an Oriental Medicine practitioner for an evaluation of your pain and to get dietary advice, but you can try eliminating the following foods to see if it helps: coffee and black tea (yes, even decaf!), alcohol, bananas, peanuts, dairy, greasy foods, pop, sugar, wheat, and spicy foods.

Environmental allergies must be controlled as much as possible, and if you see a specialist for a skin test to identify allergens, they will make specific suggestions based on the allergen. A good HEPA air filter will help substantially, and you will need one for each room. Make sure each unit is large enough to cover the needed square footage. Not all air filters are equal, so be sure to research your options. An ozonator will kill molds, but I do not suggest leaving one running while you or pets are in the room, even though some are made for that purpose. Get an ozonator that puts out enough ozone that you can "bomb" the room while you and your pets are gone. Bomb one room at a time and close the door so that you will get a high concentration. After a few hours, hold your breath and open the windows and let the room air out for a couple of minutes before you occupy the room again. You will smell ozone (like lightening) lingering, but the air is fine to breathe after just a few minutes, so don't be concerned.

Seasonal Affective Disorder (SAD) affects millions of people to one degree or another, particularly people living closer to the North or South poles where the daylight hours are shorter in winter. SAD causes symptoms such as depression, loss of energy, decreased activity, fatigue, sleeping up to four extra hours per night, irritability and crying spells, difficulty concentrating, carbohydrate cravings, and increased appetite and weight gain. Though SAD probably does not directly cause pain, many of these symptoms *can* contribute to pain eventually. For example, if increased activity helps reduce your pain but SAD keeps you from exercising, then the SAD needs to be treated in order to help reduce your pain. Most SAD patients improve when they get additional light in their retinas. Unless you sit right next to a window in your office, you are probably not getting enough light. You may be traveling to and from work in the dark much of the year. One solution is to make sure you get outside during daylight hours, possibly for a walk at your lunch hour. Another solution is to buy a therapeutic light box. Full-spectrum lights alone are not strong enough to be of therapeutic value, so you need to get a box with reflective materials capable of producing 10,000 LUX. You need to be within 24" of the box in most cases (the light box should come with instructions that tell you how close you need to be to get 10,000 LUX), and you need to have your eyes open and looking toward the box so you get the light in your retinas.

Toxic metals exposure has been implicated in pain syndromes. A hair analysis obtained through a naturopathic doctor can evaluate toxic levels of chemicals and mineral levels. If you find you have high levels of toxic metals, the doctor can help you with a detox program.

Emotional Factors

While it is important to recognize the role of stress and emotional factors in creating and perpetuating illness, unfortunately all too often patients are dismissed (or medicated) by their health care providers as "just being under stress." They depart the health care provider's office with their physical symptoms not being assessed or addressed, particularly when it comes to the symptoms of pain and depression. This seems to happen more frequently to women, but I've also had male patients who had the same experience.

Antidepressants are often prescribed, which may possibly help with the acute symptoms, but the side-effects can add to the underlying condition causing the symptoms, and a vicious cycle ensues. If you are in pain long enough, of *course* you will begin to get fatigued and depressed. If you are depressed long enough, you will probably develop pain. Anything that has gone on long enough *will* have both components.

One of the things I like most about Oriental Medicine and homeopathy is that both modalities assume you cannot separate the physical body from the emotions, and symptoms of both are used to develop a diagnosis, and are treated simultaneously. With acupuncture there are no side-effects, and response is usually rapid. With both homeopathy and herbs (Chinese or American) the wrong prescription or dosage can have side-effects, just as with Western prescription drugs, so it is important to consult with a trained professional.

If you are **angry, anxious or stressed**, chances are you are holding at least some of your body parts very tense, and developing trigger points. You may be hiking your shoulders up around your neck, tightening your forearms or abdomen, or tensing your gluteal muscles (women tense their gluteal muscles more often than men). In addition to dealing with the underlying cause of emotional factors, you will have to notice when you are tensing body parts, and keep consciously relaxing them over and over again. You are re-training yourself to not tense your muscles. Bio-feedback can help with this.

If you are experiencing an unusual desire to be alone, a disinterest in your favorite activities, a decrease in job performance, and are neglecting your appearance and hygiene, you may be suffering from **depression**. Other symptoms of depression are insomnia, loss of appetite, weight loss, impotence or a lowered libido, blurred vision, a sad mood, thoughts of suicide or death, an inability to concentrate, a poor memory, indecision, mumbled speech, and negative reactions to suggestions. No one symptom will confirm a diagnosis of depression, because there are other reasons for some of these symptoms. It is the combination of symptoms that confirms a depression diagnosis. Depression lowers your pain threshold, increases pain, and adversely affects your response to trigger point therapy. (See the section on Organ Dysfunction and Disease, **thyroid**, below, since thyroid problems can be an undiagnosed cause of depression.)

If you are angry, depressed, anxious, or stressed, you will need to address this in some manner in order to speed recovery from pain. Often people suffering from severe emotional factors, chronic fatigue and/or extreme pain lack the energy to participate in their own healing. You may have difficulty feeding yourself properly or even getting out of bed, and cannot manage even mild forms of exercise such as walking -- the very things that would help you start to feel better. You may have difficulty making it to your appointments. If this describes you, you will need to do *whatever you can* to get to the point where you can start taking better care of yourself. This may mean getting antidepressants, acupuncture, homeopathy, counseling, pain relievers, and/or doing the self-help techniques in this book. Walking and deep breathing are great tension and depression-relievers. Even walking ten minutes per day (especially outside) can be extremely beneficial. Just doing one of these things will help get you started in the right direction and improve your energy and outlook.

"Secondary Gains"

Sometimes we subconsciously get something out of being sick or in pain. For example, if you have a hard time saying "no," it is easier to excuse yourself by not feeling well, rather than having to bear the brunt of the reactions you get from people who aren't used to you refusing their requests or demands. Some people have a need to stay in pain in order to get attention. Perhaps in childhood that was the only way they could get their parent's attention and they are still using that strategy as an adult. Sometimes it's easier to focus on physical symptoms than deal with underlying anxiety and emotional problems. Some people have financial reasons for not getting well, such as disability payments or lawsuit settlements, or it may get them out of some things they don't want to do.

If you find yourself complaining about your physical symptoms but not doing anything to relieve them, you might want to ask yourself what you may be getting out of staying sick. This is not always the case, as in severe depression, but it is worth at least exploring. Chances are, if you have purchased this book, you do not have subconscious needs to stay sick or in pain, since you have already taken a step to help yourself.

Good Sport Syndrome

Many people believe in pushing through the pain -- that it will make them stronger and is beneficial. Wrong! This just aggravates existing problems and makes them harder to treat. Exercise should be comfortable, such as alternating running with walking or resting in between weight repetitions, and using weights that aren't too heavy. If you tend to overdo things, you will need to back off on your activities and add them back in slowly with the guidance of your practitioner. Returning to activities too soon or excessively will quickly wipe out your therapeutic progress.

Injuries

A healthy muscle is pliable to the touch when it is not being used, but will feel firm if called upon for action. If a muscle feels firm at rest, it is tight in an unhealthy way (even if you work-out). I like to use an analogy of a rubber band or stick. Imagine that a sudden, unexpected force is applied to the "stick," or tight muscle (such as a fall). Like a stick, the muscle will be damaged. If a sudden force is applied to a pliable muscle, or "rubberband," it will stretch with the force instead, and will be much less likely to be injured. Since latent trigger points restrict range-of-motion to some degree, and almost everyone has some latent trigger points, a muscle may be tight and restricted without you being aware of it, and can be easily injured if a sudden force is applied.

Injuries are one of the most common initiators of trigger points. **People who exercise regularly are less likely to develop trigger points** than those who exercise occasionally and overdo it. If you have an injury, begin treatment as soon as possible. Apply cold during the first 48 hours, and use some form of arnica homeopathic orally and/or topically as soon as possible. There are Chinese herb formulas for trauma that you can get from an acupuncturist or possibly a health food store. Have these available in your medicine cabinet since it may be hard for you to go to the store after you are injured, and because these work best when started immediately after the injury. See an acupuncturist or massage therapist who is experienced in working with recent injuries. You may also need to see a chiropractor, osteopathic physician, or physical therapist.

Surgeries will likely leave some amount of scar tissue, which can perpetuate trigger points in adjacent muscle fibers. **Scar tissue** can be broken up to an extent with cross-friction massage. Because this is usually fairly painful, I only work on scars for a few minutes each appointment, and I warn the patient that it will be painful but that I won't do it for more than a few minutes. Most patients will not work on their own scars vigorously enough due to the pain level. Acupuncture can treat scar tissue and help eliminate the pain from trigger points around the area. I recommend using both cross-friction massage and acupuncture as part of the treatment protocol, rather than just one or the other.

Mechanical Stresses

Chronic mechanical stresses are one of the most common causes of trigger point activation and perpetuation, and are nearly always correctable. A **skeletal asymmetry**, including an anatomically shorter leg and a small hemipelvis (either the right or left half of the pelvis) can be corrected with shoe lifts and butt lifts. [NOTE: In this book, reference to a "shorter leg" refers to a *true* anatomical leg length inequality where the bones are shorter on one side, rather than the "shorter leg" caused by a spinal mis-alignment, which is a term chiropractors use.] A **skeletal disproportion**, such as a long second toe can be corrected with shoe orthotics, and short upper arms can be corrected with ergonomically correct furniture. Vertebral subluxation and other bones-out-alignment can be adjusted by a chiropractor or osteopathic physician, especially if the muscles are also first relaxed by an acupuncturist or massage therapist. Your physical therapist may be trained in manipulations.

Wearing appropriate shoes can help relieve symptoms in your entire body (see "Abuse of Muscles," below). **Orthotics** can help even more. My favorite non-corrective orthotics are the Superfeet brand. They have a deep heel cup which helps prevent pronation (more weight on the inside of your foot) and supination (more weight on the outside of the foot), and they have excellent arch support. Superfeet has a variety of models, including cheaper non-custom "Trim-to-Fit" footbeds, and moderately-priced custom molded footbeds to provide support in a variety of footwear. See Superfeet.com to learn more about their products. If you find you need corrective orthotics, you will need to see a podiatrist. If you decide to get custom orthotics, be sure to work on your trigger points first, because as the muscles relax you will stand differently and the orthotics need to be formed for the corrected stance.

Misfitting furniture is a major cause of muscular pain, particularly in the work place. There are companies that specialize in coming into your work place and correcting your office arrangement, and fitting you for furniture that fits your body. Your employer may balk at the cost, but if they don't change your misfitting furniture, they will end up paying for it in lost work time and worker's compensation claims.

I see a lot of what I call "mouse injuries" -- arm and shoulder pain due to using a computer mouse for extended periods of time without proper arm support. The keyboard should be kept as close to lap level as possible. When not using your computer, your elbows and forearms should rest evenly on either your work surface or armrests of the proper height. Your computer screen should be directly in front of you with the middle of the screen slightly below eye level, and the copy attached to the side of the screen, so that you may look directly forward as much as possible. Your knees should fit under your desk, and the chair needs to be close enough that you can lean against your backrest. A good chair will have a backrest with a slope of 25 to 30-degrees back from the vertical which supports both the lumbar area and the mid-back. The seat should be low enough that your feet rest flat on the floor without compression of the thigh by the front edge of the seat, high enough that not all the pressure is put on the buttocks, and slightly hollowed out to accommodate the buttocks. The armrests must be high enough to provide support for the elbows without having to lean to the side, but not so high as to cause the shoulders to hike up. The upholstery needs to be firm and casters should be avoided. I highly recommend headsets for phones to solve neck and back pain.

A lumbar support helps correct round-shouldered posture. Most chiropractic offices carry lumbar supports of varying thickness. I recommend getting one for the car (most car seats actually *curve the wrong way* in the lumbar area) and your favorite seat at home, and investing in a good chair for the office, even if your employer won't. Try to avoid sitting in or on anything without back support, which causes you to sit with your shoulders and upper back slumped forward. When going to sporting events, picnics, or other places you won't have a back support, bring a *Crazy Creek Chair*™ (or something similar) to provide at least some support. You can get one through most of the major sporting goods suppliers for about $49, a good investment in your back, and they are very lightweight for carrying. Or consider a lightweight collapsible chair, also available at sporting goods stores.

Sleeping in a sagging bed can cause back and hip problems. (See the section on Sleep Problems below).

But properly fitting furniture won't help as much if you are not also conscientious of avoiding **poor posture**. If you slouch at your desk or on your couch at home, or read in bed, for example, your muscles will suffer. **Abuse of muscles** includes poor body mechanics (i.e., lifting improperly), long periods of immobility (i.e., sitting at a desk without a break), repetitive movements (i.e., computer use), holding your body in an awkward position for long periods (i.e., dentists and mechanics), and excessively quick and jerky movements (i.e., sports). Learn to lift properly and take frequent breaks from anything you must do for long time periods.

If you have a habit of immobilizing your muscles to protect against pain, you will need to start gently increasing your range of motion as you inactivate trigger points. Don't keep stressing the muscles to see if it still hurts or to demonstrate to your treating professionals where you have to move it to in order to get it to hurt -- if you keep repeating this motion, you will just keep the trigger points activated.

Be sure to sit while putting clothing on your lower body. Don't wear high heels or cowboy boots. If you carry a purse, get a strap long enough that you can wear it diagonally across your body, rather than over one shoulder. If you use a day pack, put the straps over both shoulders. Without realizing it, you are hiking up one shoulder at least a little to keep the straps from slipping off no matter *how* light your purse or pack may be. Notice whether you hold your shoulders up or are tightening muscles such as your butt, arms, or abdomen when you are under stress. You will need to re-train yourself to break this habit.

If you are clenching your jaw or grinding your teeth, see a dentist for help. The soft plastic bite splints found over-the-counter in pharmacies are too soft and do not help temporomandibular joint dysfunction. You need to be fitted by your dentist for a hard, slippery acrylic night guard.

Constricting clothing can lead to muscular problems. My rule of thumb is, if the clothing item leaves an elastic mark or indentation in the skin, it is too tight and is cutting off proper circulation. Check your bras, socks, ties, and belts to see if they are too tight.

Be sure to check muscles listed in the muscle chapters that can cause "satellite trigger points," since this is one perpetuating cause. For example, if you find trigger points in the abdominal muscles but trigger points quickly recur, check the paraspinal muscles also, because trigger points there can refer to the abdominal area and cause trigger points to be reactivated.

Nutritional Problems and Diet

Doctors Travell and Simons found that almost half of their patients required treatment for **vitamin inadequacies** to obtain lasting relief from the pain and dysfunction of trigger points, and thought it was one of the most important perpetuating factors to address. They found **the most important were the water-soluble vitamins B-1, B-6, B-12, folic acid, vitamin C, and the minerals calcium, magnesium, iron and potassium**. Other researchers have now added **vitamin D** to that list.

The more deficient in nutrients you are, the more symptoms you will have, and your trigger points and nervous system will be more hyper-irritable. Even if a blood test determines you are at the low end of the normal range, you may still need more of a nutrient, since your body will pull nutrients from the tissues before it will allow a decrease in the blood levels. Several factors may lead to nutrient insufficiency:

- An inadequate intake of a nutrient

- Impaired nutrient absorption
- Inadequate nutrient utilization
- An increased need by the body
- A nutrient leaving the body too quickly
- A nutrient being destroyed within the body too quickly

You may be in a **high risk group** if you are: elderly, pregnant or nursing, an alcoholic or other drug user, poor, depressed, or seriously ill. If you tend to diet by leaving out important food groups, or have an eating disorder, you will also deplete yourself of necessary nutrients.

- Even if you have a fairly healthy diet, because our soils have been depleted in nutrients from too frequent crop-rotations, chemical fertilizers, and long shipping distances, our food does not provide all the nutrition we require. In addition, many of us don't have a very balanced diet, and processed foods do not contain as much nutrition as fresh-prepared. Most people need to take some kind of **multi-supplement** to ensure proper nutrition, especially if you fall into one of the high risk groups mentioned above. Because some vitamins require the presence of other vitamins, a good multi-supplement ensures the needed combination is present. Be sure to check the label to make sure there are adequate minerals in a multi -- you may need to also take a multi-mineral. Improving your nutrient intake to see if it improves your symptoms is an easy and relatively inexpensive therapy to try. Take your vitamins with food, since some need to bind with substances found in food in order to be absorbed.

    Building up sufficient levels of vitamin B-12, vitamin D, and iron may take several months; don't get discouraged if you don't see immediate results, though you may start gradually feeling better within a few weeks from taking multivitamin and multimineral supplements.

- You may still need to be tested by a health care provider for inadequacies, since some people are not able to absorb certain nutrients, and need to have them injected or mega-dosed. For example, some people cannot absorb B-12, and need to get intramuscular injections to provide that necessary vitamin.

- **Take your vitamins and herbs when you are *not* sick** -- the germs also like the vitamins and herbs and they will get stronger. See the section above on Acute or Chronic Viral, Bacterial, and Parasitic Infections for suggestions on how to head off illness. Once all symptoms have abated, you may switch back to your regular vitamins and herbs.

- How well your **digestive system** is functioning is also a factor. If you are not digesting well, you do not have enough enzymes or possibly hydrochloric acid to break down food properly. Taking digestive enzymes or hydrochloric acid for long periods is not a good solution, because they will take over the natural function of your body. Supplementation can be used in the short term, but you need to repair the body's natural function so it can perform its own job properly. **Digestive problems** can be addressed with the help of an acupuncturist, herbalist, or naturopath. They can give you dietary recommendations based on your unique set of health problems and constitution, and prescribe herbs to re-balance your systems.

- It is a common mis-conception that raw foods and whole grains are the healthiest way to eat. It is actually better to **cook your food** (not overcook!) in order to start the chemical breakdown process, so your digestive system doesn't have to work as hard. If you are having trouble digesting, white rice and bread are easier to digest than whole grains. Soups are nutritious and easy to digest.

- **Fasting** is hard on the digestive system. If you want to do a cleanse, use herbs and psyllium, but don't stop eating.

- Most people should not be strict vegetarians. At the very least you should eat organic eggs for a **high-quality protein** source. Most vegetarians are not very good about combining foods, and even if they are, most still seem to feel better when they add high-quality animal protein back into their diet. Plant sources contain mainly the pyridoxol form of B-6, but animal sources contain both the pyridoxal and pyridoxamine forms of B-6, and are less susceptible to the loss of the vitamin due to cooking or preserving. B-12 is *only* found in animal proteins, including dairy products. Brewer's yeast does not contain B-12, unless the yeast is grown on a special B-12-containing substrate.

- If you have **chronic diarrhea**, you will not retain food long enough in the intestines to absorb nutrients. You will need to identify and eliminate the source of diarrhea. Acupuncture, herbs, and dietary changes can often successfully address this problem.

- Excess **caffeine** increases muscle tension and trigger point irritability, leading to increased pain. Dr.'s Travell and Simons state that "... caffeine has long been known to cause a persistent contracture, or caffeine rigor, of muscle fibers. This rigor is due to enhancement by caffeine of the release of calcium from the sarcoplasmic reticulum and to interference with the rebinding of calcium ions by the sarcoplasmic reticulum." They found that caffeine in excess of 150 mg daily (more than two eight-ounce cups of regular coffee) would lead to caffeine rigor. Based on my clinical experience, some people can't even consume 150 mg without aggravating their pain. In counting your daily intake, be sure to count any caffeine in the drugs you are taking, and remember that espresso and similar drinks will have far greater amounts of caffeine. There are websites that list caffeine amounts for foods and beverages.

- **Alcohol** aggravates trigger points by decreasing serum and tissue folate levels. It increases the body's need for vitamin C, while decreasing the body's ability to absorb it. **Tobacco** also increases the need for vitamin C. In Chinese Medicine, caffeine and alcohol are said to be very "qi stagnating." **Marijuana** is very stagnating also, and stays in your system for about three months after smoking it. Stagnation is one cause of pain, therefore using any of the above substances will increase your pain level.

Copyright © 2024 Valerie DeLaune, LAc

- Eliminating foods and beverages that aggravate your condition (such as allergins, coffee, and alcohol) may not be enough, if the underlying condition that was caused by the food has not been resolved. For example, if you have been eating damp-producing foods (like dairy and peanut butter) which has led to dampness in the muscles (as in fibromyalgia), even if you stop ingesting the food or beverage you still have dampness in the muscles that must be eliminated. Plan on avoiding the necessary foods for two months minimum *in conjunction* with acupuncture and/or herbs and other supplements, in order to determine whether eliminating the food is helpful. Many people will stop ingesting a food or drink for one week, decide it hasn't made a difference, and then re-start their regular diet. Or the food or beverage is so important to them that they'd rather have pain and other medical conditions, than give the substance up. Reaching a conclusion after one week is one way to justify continuing to ingest the substance.

- **Herbs** should be taken with the advice of a qualified practitioner. I've seen many people who have injured their digestive systems by taking too many herbs, or herbs that are improper for their conditions and constitution. What may be the correct herb for a friend or a family member may not be the correct herb for you, so seek professional advice.

- Room-temperature **water** is better than cold drinks -- if you drink something cold, your stomach has to work harder to warm it up, and it taxes the digestive system. Drink about two quarts per day, or more if you have a larger body mass or sweat a lot. A general rule of thumb for kids and adults weighing more than 100 pounds is your body weight multiplied by the number of ounces (i.e., 140 lbs. = 70 ounces). Drink at least one extra quart per day if it is very hot out, and extra water during and immediately after a work-out. If you drink *too* much water, you can deplete Vitamin B-1 (thiamine). Thirst is not necessarily a good indicator of whether or not you are dehydrated. Your urine should be a light yellow, unless you have just taken a multivitamin or B-vitamin supplement.

- **Don't drink distilled water**, because you need the minerals found in non-distilled water. If you drink bottled water, make sure you know its source, and that it is not distilled. This industry is not currently regulated, so you may need to do some research on the company.

Vitamins

- **Vitamin C** reduces post-exercise soreness and corrects the capillary fragility which leads to easy bruising. (Hint: if you don't remember how you got a bruise, you are likely bruising too easily.) It is essential for collagen formation (connective tissue) and forming bones. Vitamin C is required for synthesis of the neurotransmitters norepinephrine and serotonin, is needed for your body's response to stress, is important for immune system function, and decreases the irritability of trigger points caused by infection.

Too *much* Vitamin C can lead to watery diarrhea or non-specific urethritis. However, Vitamin C helps terminate diarrhea due to food allergies. Vitamin C daily doses above 400mg are not used by the body, and 1000mg/day increases the risk of kidney stone formation, so mega-dosing with Vitamin C is not necessary nor recommended. Women taking estrogen or oral contraceptives may need 500mg/day.

Vitamin C is likely to be deficient in smokers, alcoholics, older people (the presence of Vitamin C in the tissues decreases with age), infants fed primarily on cows' milk (usually between the ages of 6-12 months), people with chronic diarrhea, psychiatric patients, and fad dieters. Initial symptoms of deficiency include weakness, lethargy, irritability, vague aching pains in the joints and muscles, easy bruising, and possibly weight loss. In severe cases of Vitamin C deficiency (scurvy), the gums become red, swollen, bleed easily, and teeth may become loose and fall out.

Do not take Vitamin C with antacids; since Vitamin C is ascorbic acid, and the purpose of an antacid is to neutralize acid, antacids will neutralize Vitamin C and make it ineffective. Food sources include citrus fruits and *fresh* juices, *raw* broccoli, *raw* Brussels sprouts, collard, kale, turnip greens, guava, *raw* sweet peppers, cabbage, and potatoes

- **Taking too many vitamins A, D, and E, and folic acid** can cause symptoms similar to deficiencies, so don't mega-dose on those supplements unless a health care provider has determined your condition warrants it.

- **Thiamine (Vitamin B-1)** is essential for normal nerve function and energy production within muscle cells. Diminished pain and temperature sensitivity and an inability to detect vibrations indicate you are low in thiamine. You may also possibly experience calf cramping at night, slight sweating, constipation, and fatigue. B-1 is needed for proper thyroid hormone levels (see the section on Organ Dysfunction and Disease below). Abuse of alcohol reduces thiamine absorption, and absorption is further reduced if liver disease is also present. The tannin in black tea, antacid use, and a magnesium deficiency can also prevent the absorption of thiamine. Thiamine can be destroyed by processing foods, and by heating them to temperatures above 212º F (100º C). Thiamine is excreted too rapidly when taking diuretics or drinking too much water. Lean pork, kidney, liver, beef, eggs, fish, beans, nuts, and some whole grain cereals (if the hull and germ are present) are good sources of thiamine.

- **Pyridoxine (Vitamin B-6)** is important for nerve function, energy metabolism, amino acid metabolism, and synthesis of neurotransmitters including norepinephrine and serotonin, which strongly influence pain perception. Deficiency of B-6 results in anemia, reduced absorption and storage of B-12, increased excretion of Vitamin C, blocked synthesis of niacin, and can lead to a hormonal imbalance. Deficiency of B-6 will manifest as symptoms of one of the other B-vitamins, since B-6 is needed in order for all the others to perform their functions. The need for B-6 increases with age and increased protein consumption. Tropical sprue and alcohol use interfere with its absorption. Use of **oral contraceptives** increases your requirement for B-6, and impairs glucose tolerance. This can lead to depression if you don't supplement with B-6, particularly if you already have a history of depression. Corticosteroid use, excessive alcohol use, pregnancy and lactation, antitubercular drugs, uremia, and hyperthyroidism also increase the need for B-6. Sources of B-6 include liver, kidney, chicken (white meat), halibut, tuna, English walnuts, soybean flour, navy beans, bananas, and avocados. There is also some amount of B-6 present in yeast, lean beef, egg yolk, and whole wheat.

- **Cobalamin (Vitamin B-12) and Folic Acid** need to be taken together to form erythrocytes (a type of red blood cell) and rapidly dividing cells such as those found in the gastrointestinal tract, and for fatty acid synthesis used in the formation of parts of certain nerve fibers. B-12 is needed for both fat and carbohydrate metabolism. A deficiency can result in **pernicious (megaloblastic) anemia**, which reduces oxygen coming to the site of the trigger point, adding to the dysfunctional cycle and increasing pain. A deficiency of B-12 may also cause symptoms such as non-specific depression, fatigue, an exaggerated startle reaction to noise or touch, and an increased susceptibility to trigger points. B-12 is only found in animal products or supplements. Several drugs may impair the absorption of B-12, as can mega-doses of Vitamin C for long periods of time.

- A **folate deficiency** (also known as **folic acid** when in the synthetic form) can cause you to be fatigued easily, sleep poorly, and feel discouraged and depressed. It can cause "restless legs," diffuse muscular pain, diarrhea, a loss of sensation in the extremities, and you may feel cold frequently, along with a slightly lower basal body temperature than the "normal" 98.6º F (37º C). Folic acid deficiency is very prevalent and can lead to **megaloblastic anemia**. In the U.S., studies have shown that at least 15% of Caucasians are deficient, while at least 30% of African-Americans and Latinos are deficient. At least half of Canadians eat less than the dietary recommendation. Part of the problem is that 50-95% of the folate content of foods may be destroyed in food processing and preparation, so even if you eat folate sources, you may not be receiving the benefit. A necessary conversion in the digestive system is inhibited by peas, beans, citrus fruits, acidic foods, and antacids, so eat these separately from your folic acid sources. The best sources of folate are leafy vegetables, yeast, organ meat, fruit, and lightly cooked vegetables such as broccoli and asparagus. You are at greatest risk for folate deficiency if you are elderly, have a bowel disorder, are pregnant or lactating, or use drugs and alcohol regularly. Certain other drugs will also deplete folate, such as anti-inflammatories (including aspirin), diuretics, estrogens (such as birth control pills), and anti-convulsants. You must also have adequate B-12 intake in order to absorb folic acid, plus only taking one of these can mask a severe deficiency in the other.

- **Vitamin D** is required for both the absorption and the utilization of calcium and phosphorus. It is necessary for growth and thyroid function, it protects against muscle weakness, and helps regulate the heartbeat. It is important for the prevention of cancer, osteoarthritis, osteoporosis, and calcium deficiency. A mild deficiency of vitamin D may manifest as a loss of appetite, a burning sensation in the mouth and throat, diarrhea, insomnia, visual problems, and weight loss. It has been estimated that close to 90% of patients with chronic musculoskeletal pain may have a vitamin D deficiency.

Vitamin D-3 is synthesized by the skin when exposed to the sun's UV rays. Unfortunately, many people don't get enough sun exposure, especially if they live at latitudes or in climates with little sun available during the winter months. Exposing your face and arms to the sun for 15 minutes three times per week will ensure that your body synthesizes an adequate amount of vitamin D. Because the amount of exposure needed varies from person to person and also depends on geographical location, you will need to do some personal research and perhaps consult with a dermatologist to determine the proper amount for you. Food sources of vitamin D include salmon, halibut, sardines, tuna, and eggs. Other sources include dairy products, dandelion greens, liver, oatmeal, and sweet potatoes. If you take supplements, look for the D-3 form, or fish oil capsules.

Minerals

Inadequate salt, calcium/magnesium, or potassium can lead to **muscle cramping**.

- Do not entirely eliminate **salt** from your diet, especially if you sweat. You do need some salt in your diet (unless you have been instructed otherwise by your health care provider for certain medical conditions), though you don't want to overdo it either.

- **Calcium, magnesium, potassium, and iron** are needed for proper muscle function. Iron is required for oxygen transport to the muscle fibers. Calcium is essential for releasing acetylcholine at the nerve terminal, and both calcium and magnesium are needed for the contracting mechanism of the muscle fiber. Potassium is needed to get the muscle fiber quickly ready for its next contraction. Deficiency of these minerals increases the irritability of trigger points. Calcium, magnesium, and potassium should be taken together, because an increase in one can deplete the others. Also needed for good health but not as important for muscle function are zinc, iodine, copper, manganese, chromium, selenium, and molybdenum.

  It is especially important to take **calcium** for at least a few years prior to menopause to help prevent osteoporosis. Vitamin D is needed for calcium uptake. Food sources of calcium include dairy (though this is not recommended for people with damp conditions, such as fibromyalgia), salmon, sardines, seafood, green leafy vegetables, almonds, asparagus, blackstrap molasses, brewer's yeast, broccoli, cabbage, carob, collards, dandelion greens, figs, filberts, kale, kelp, mustard greens, oats, parsley, prunes, sesame seeds, tofu, turnip greens, and whey.

- Do not take Tums or other **antacids** as a source of **calcium**. Stomach acid is needed for the uptake of calcium, but an antacid neutralizes stomach acid. So even if there is calcium present, it cannot be used. If you must take an antacid, take it several hours apart from your calcium/magnesium supplement so you will maximize your mineral uptake. **Calcium channel blockers** prescribed for high blood pressure inhibit the uptake of calcium into the sarcoplasmic reticulum of vascular smooth muscles and cardiac muscles. Since this is likely also true for skeletal muscles, calcium channel blockers would also make trigger points worse, and more difficult to treat. See your health care provider to find out if you can switch to a different medication. Consider treating the underlying causes of hypertension with acupuncture, diet changes, exercise, or whatever is appropriate to your particular set of circumstances.

- **Magnesium deficiency** is less likely to occur as a result of an inadequate dietary intake in a healthy diet as it is to malabsorption, malnutrition, kidney disease, or fluid and electrolyte loss. Magnesium is depleted after strenuous physical exercise, but proper amounts of exercise coupled with an adequate intake of magnesium improves the efficiency of cellular metabolism and improves cardio-respiratory performance. Consumption of alcohol, the use of diuretics, chronic diarrhea, consumption of fluoride, and high amounts of zinc and Vitamin D increase the body's need for magnesium.

    Magnesium is found in most foods, especially dairy products (though this is not recommended for people with damp conditions, such as fibromyalgia), fish, meat, seafood, apples, apricots, avocados, bananas, blackstrap molasses, brewer's yeast, brown rice, figs, garlic, kelp, lima beans, millet, nuts, peaches, black-eyes peas, salmon, sesame seeds, tofu, green leafy vegetable, wheat, and whole grains.

- A diet high in fats, refined sugars, and too much salt causes **potassium deficiency**, as does the use of laxatives and some diuretics. Diarrhea will also deplete potassium. If you suffer from urinary frequency, particularly if your urine is clear rather than light yellow, try taking potassium. Frequent urination causes potassium deficiency, and potassium deficiency may cause frequent urination, and a cycle of depletion ensues. Food sources of potassium include fruit (especially bananas and citrus fruits), potatoes, green leafy vegetables, wheat germ, beans, lentils, nuts, dates, and prunes.

- **Iron deficiency** can lead to **anemia**, and is usually caused by excessive blood loss from a heavy menses, hemorrhoids, intestinal bleeding, donating blood too often, or ulcers. Iron deficiency can also be caused by a long-term illness, prolonged use of antacids, poor digestion, excess coffee or black tea consumption, or the chronic use of NSAID's (non-steroidal anti-inflammatory drugs, such as ibuprofen). Calcium in milk, cheese, or as a supplement can impair absorption of iron, therefore you should take your calcium supplement separately. Do not take an iron supplement if you have an infection or cancer. The body stores it in order to withhold it from bacteria, and in the case of cancer, it may suppress the cancer-killing function of certain cells.

    Early symptoms of iron deficiency include impaired work performance, fatigue, reduced endurance, and an inability to stay warm when exposed to a moderately cold environment. 9-11% of menstruating females in the U.S. are iron deficient, and the world-wide prevalence is about 15%. Iron is best absorbed with Vitamin C. Generally food sources are adequate for improving iron levels for most people. Good sources of iron include eggs, fish, liver, meat, poultry, green leafy vegetables, whole grains, almonds, avocados, beets, blackstrap molasses, brewer's yeast, dates, egg yolks, kelp, kidney and lima beans, lentils, millet, parsley, peaches, pears, dried prunes, pumpkin, raisins, rice and wheat bran, sesame seeds, and soybeans.

One of my favorite books is "*Prescription for Nutritional Healing*" by James F. Balch, M.D., and Phyllis A. Balch, C.N.C.. It has a comprehensive list of vitamins, minerals, amino acids, antioxidants, and enzymes, and food sources for each. It has sections on common disorders listing supplements needed to treat each condition, and helpful hints.

Hormonal Changes

Women are more likely than men to develop trigger points. I have noticed this is particularly true in **menopausal** women. Some teenagers (of both sexes) going through **puberty** also seem to have a tendency to develop trigger points, leading me to believe there is a connection between hormonal changes and one potential cause of trigger points.

Organ Dysfunction and Disease

Thyroid

Both **thyroid inadequacy** (also known as hypometabolism or subclinical hypothyroidism) and **hypothyroidism** will cause and perpetuate trigger points. Hypothyroid patients may experience early morning stiffness, and pain and weakness of the shoulder girdle. Both thyroid inadequacy and hypothyroidism will produce symptoms of cold (and sometimes heat) intolerance, cold hands and feet, muscle aches and pains especially with cold rainy weather, constipation, menstrual problems, weight gain, dry skin, and fatigue and lethargy. Muscles feel rather hard to the touch, and even if a patient is on a thyroid supplement, I've noticed they are still somewhat prone to trigger points, since it is hard to fine-tune the medication exactly to the amount your body would produce if you still had a healthy thyroid organ. Some studies report the prevalence of subclinical hypothyroidism to be as high as 17% in women and 7% in men. Occasionally patients with inadequate metabolism may be thin, nervous, and hyperactive, which may result in a health care provider failing to consider subclinical hypothyroidism.

Patients with low thyroid function may be **low in thiamine (Vitamin B-1)**. Before starting on thyroid medication, try supplementing with thiamine to see if that corrects your thyroid hormone levels. If you are already on thyroid medication and you start taking B-1, you may start exhibiting symptoms of *hyper*thyroidism, and your medication dosage needs to be adjusted. If you are low in B-1 at the time of starting thyroid medication, you may develop symptoms of acute thiamine deficiency, which may be misinterpreted as an intolerance to the medication. After the B-1 deficiency is corrected, you will likely tolerate the medication. You will need to supplement with B-1 prior to and during thyroid hormone therapy to avoid a deficiency. Total body potassium is low in hypothyroidism, and high in hyperthyroidism, so you may need to adjust your potassium intake also.

Smoking impairs the action of thyroid hormone and will make any related symptoms worse. Several pharmaceutical drugs can also affect thyroid hormone levels, such as lithium, anti-convulsants, those that contain iodine, and glucocorticoid steroids, so check with your pharmacist if you have been diagnosed with hypothyroidism and are taking another medication.

A simple **home test** to check your thyroid function is to place a thermometer in your armpit for 10 minutes upon waking but before getting out of bed. Normal underarm temperature for men and post-menopausal women is 98º F (36.7º C). If you are still menstruating your temperature should be around 97.5º F (36.4º C) prior to ovulation, and 98.5º F (36.9º C) following ovulation. If your temperature is lower than this, you will want to check with your health care provider. Often health care providers will only initially test the TSH level, which may still be normal if you have hypometabolism rather than hypothyroidism. A radioimmunoassay measures T3 and T4 levels, and gives a more complete picture of the thyroid function.

If you are suffering from depression, be sure to insist that your thyroid levels are tested before starting on anti-depressant medication. I've had more than one patient (especially men) where hypothyroidism was discovered only after they had been medicated for some time.

Hypoglycemia

Both **postprandial (reactive) and fasting hypoglycemia** cause and perpetuate trigger points, and make trigger points more difficult to treat. Symptoms of both are sweating, trembling and shakiness, increased heart rate, and anxiety. Activation of trigger points in the *sternocleidomastoid* muscle by a hypoglycemic reaction may lead to dizziness and headaches. If allowed to progress, symptoms can include visual disturbances, restlessness, and impaired speech and thinking. Missing or delaying a meal does not cause hypoglycemia in a healthy person. A hypoglycemic reaction to a delayed meal usually indicates a problem with the liver, adrenal glands, or pituitary gland. Postprandial hypoglycemia usually occurs two to three hours after eating a meal rich in carbohydrates, and is most like to occur when you are under high stress.

Causes will need to be identified and addressed, if possible. Symptoms will be relieved by eating smaller, more frequent meals with fewer carbohydrates, more protein, and some fat. Avoid all caffeine, alcohol, and tobacco (even second-hand smoke). If you are waking with headaches or pain or having trouble sleeping, try eating a small snack or drink a little juice before bedtime to see if it relieves your symptoms; it usually helps. Acupuncture is quite successful in stabilizing blood sugar.

Gout

Gout will aggravate trigger points and make them difficult to treat. Doctors Travell and Simons recommend keeping the gout under control and taking Vitamin C, and then subsequent treatment of trigger points will be more effective.

Sleep Problems

Pain can interrupt sleep, and interrupted sleep can perpetuate trigger points. It is useful to know whether your sleep was interrupted before your pain started, or whether your sleep was sound and restful. If your sleep was poor prior to the pain, then there is another underlying factor which needs to be addressed to help solve the problem.

Be sure you are not sleeping poorly due to being **too warm or too cold**. If you have

problems falling asleep, try improving your nutrition and your water intake first. Take a calcium/magnesium supplement before bedtime. If you are **waking easily due to noise**, try Mack's™ soft silicon earplugs (my favorite), and try breathing deeply until you fall back to sleep. If you can't stop thinking, you sleep lightly and wake frequently, you wake early and can't fall back to sleep, are menopausal, and/or have vivid and disturbing dreams, try acupuncture and Chinese herbs.

Even if you only drink **caffeine** in the morning, it still disturbs your nighttime sleep pattern, as does **alcohol**. If you choose to give up caffeine, it will take about two weeks before your energy starts to even out and you don't feel like you have to use it to get going in the morning. **Computer use in the evening** stimulates the brain and makes it hard to fall asleep and sleep restfully. If **urinary frequency** is disturbing your sleep, try acupuncture and herbs, and increasing your potassium intake.

Consider whether your **adrenal glands** could be excreting too much cortisol (the "stress hormone"). If you are continually stressed, or if you are pushing yourself too hard and push through fatigue instead of resting or taking a nap, you will excrete more cortisol and have more difficulty sleeping at night. A Naturopathic doctor can administer a saliva test for adrenal function.

Make sure you are not being exposed to **allergens** at night. Get inexpensive soft plastic covers for your pillows and mattress, since many people are allergic to mites, and they live in your bedding. If you have a down comforter or pillow, you may be allergic to the feathers, even if you are not exhibiting classic allergic symptoms, such as sneezing and itchy eyes.

Beds that are too soft can cause a lot of muscular problems, and you may not know it is too soft. Patients usually insist their mattress is firm enough, but when queried further, will admit that sleeping on a mat on the floor gives them relief when the pain is particularly bad. If this is the case, your mattress is not firm enough, no matter how much money you spent on it or how well it worked for someone else. Different people have needs for different kinds of mattresses. An all-cotton futon is very firm, and may be best for some people. The "Sleep Number" bed allows you to change the firmness and some models have an option to control firmness separately for each side of the bed. A lot of people like memory foam beds, but I personally find them too soft. Try putting some camp mats on the floor and sleeping on them for a week. If you feel better, it is time for a new, firmer mattress. Mattresses really only last about five to seven years, and should then be replaced. Some furniture stores will let you try a mattress out for a time period before making a final decision. Be sure you have a **pillow** that keeps your head in line with your spine -- not too high or too low. Sleeping on the couch should definitely be avoided.

If pain disturbs you at night, I sometimes suggest to patients that they keep their self-help ball collection by their bed so that if they wake they can work on their trigger points, and hopefully fall back to sleep once the pain is reduced. The danger in this is that *you have to be sure you don't fall asleep on the ball*! It will cut off the circulation for too long, and make the trigger points worse. It is an easy thing to do when you are fatigued and in pain, and suddenly the pain is reduced or gone, so don't use the ball in bed unless you are sure you will not fall asleep on it.

Spinal Mis-alignments and Other Problems

Vertebrae may be out-of-alignment, and need to be adjusted by a chiropractor or osteopathic physician, or mobilized by a physical therapist. Usually there is also a muscular component that caused the mis-alignment to begin with, so a combined approach of skeletal mobilization and massage or acupuncture is probably necessary for lasting relief. A chiropractor or osteopathic physician will likely take x-rays at the initial visit to evaluate your spine. If you have already had x-rays taken, bring them with you to the visit so you can avoid duplicating x-rays.

Herniated and bulging disks may be very successfully treated with acupuncture (especially Plum Blossom technique), but if you don't get some relief fairly quickly, you may want to consider surgery if you have insurance. Spinal surgery has gotten so sophisticated that many surgeries are fairly minor procedures that have you back on your feet the next day. If you have **stenosis** (a narrowing of the central spinal cord canal or the holes the nerves come out of) acupuncture will help with pain, but not the stenosis, so surgery is probably the best option. With any surgery there is a certain amount of risk, so be sure to discuss this with your operating physician, and make sure you understand the procedure. If you are still unsure, get a second opinion from another surgeon. Disc problems and stenosis need to be confirmed with an MRI.

Bone spurs and narrowed disc spaces can cause pain. But in a random sample of the population you will find many people with bone spurs and narrowed disc spaces with no pain, and many people with pain and no bone spurs or narrowed disc spaces, so don't assume these are causing your problems, even if a health care provider has made this assumption.

I always start with the assumption that trigger points are at least part of the problem, if not all of the problem, and treat accordingly. If a patient doesn't receive some relief fairly quickly, then I know there may be something else going on and I refer them to someone who can evaluate them with an x-ray or MRI.

If you have had surgery and your pain continues, trigger points are the likely culprit, and need to be treated for lasting relief. If you still do not get relief, there is a possibility the pain is due to scar tissue from the surgery compressing a nerve root, so you will need to check with your health care provider.

Laboratory Tests

Laboratory tests may be necessary to help diagnose some of the systemic perpetuating factors. With blood chemistry profiles, an elevated erythrocyte sedimentation rate (**SED Rate**) may indicate a chronic bacterial infection, polymyositis, polymyalgia rheumatica, rheumatoid arthritis, or cancer. A decreased **erythrocyte count** and/or **low hemoglobin** points to anemia. A mean corpuscular volume (**MCV**) of over 92fl indicates the likelihood of a folate or B-12 deficiency. **Eosinophilia** may indicate an allergy or intestinal parasitic infection. An increase in **monocytes** can indicate low thyroid function, infectious mononucleosis, or an acute viral infection. Increased serum **cholesterol** can be caused by a problem with low thyroid function, and a low serum cholesterol can indicate folate deficiency. High **uric acid** levels indicate hyperuricemia and possibly gout.

Iron deficiency is detected by checking the **serum ferritin** level. A **fasting blood test** is used to diagnose hypoglycemia, and an additional **glucose tolerance test** or a 2-hour postprandial blood glucose test may be used to rule out diabetes. (Measurement of **sensory**

nerve conduction velocities can help diagnose diabetic neuropathy.) A low serum total calcium suggests a calcium deficiency, but for an accurate assessment of the available calcium, a **serum ionized calcium** test needs to be performed. **Potassium** levels can be checked with a serum potassium test.

Blood tests can determine **serum levels of Vitamins B-1, B-6, B-12, folic acid, and Vitamins C and D.** Any values in the lower 25% of the normal range or below would indicate that supplementation would be helpful in the treatment of trigger points. Remember that even if serum levels of vitamins and minerals are normal, you may still wish to use supplements since tissue supplies will drop before the body allows serum levels in the blood to drop.

See the above section on Nutritional Problems for comments on the digestive system and vitamin and mineral sources. See the above section on Organ Dysfunction and Disease for a discussion of thyroid function tests. A hair analysis can detect high levels of toxic metals exposure and deficiencies in minerals. A naturopathic doctor can perform **blood tests for food allergies**. Stool samples will reveal if **parasites** are a problem.

Other Books by the Author

Pain Relief with Trigger Point Self Help, DeLaune, Valerie LAc

On-line format (2004, revised 2012, 2017). A multimedia membership website for pain relief, appropriate for both practitioners and the lay public. It contains information on the causes and locations of trigger points for the entire body, along with hundreds of color photos with overlays of common pain referral patterns, and 144 video clips of self-help techniques for applying pressure to trigger points and performing stretches. A search feature allows you to search for your related medical conditions. Because the website navigates in your web browser, it is easy to locate the source of your pain, and move from one relevant chapter to the next.

It contains introductory chapters on the physiology and characteristics of trigger points, and a comprehensive chapter on all of the perpetuating factors that can cause and keep trigger points activated, along with solutions. Perpetuating factors include poor ergonomics and poorly-designed furniture, clothing problems, inadequate nutrition, inadequate water, improper diet, injuries, spinal and skeletal factors, sleep problems, emotional factors, allergies, hormonal imbalances, organ dysfunction or disease, and acute or chronic viral, bacterial, or parasitic infections. For more information on how to subscribe to this website, and for additional resources, go to "http://triggerpointrelief.net/"

Other Titles by Valerie DeLaune, LAc

Trigger Point Therapy Workbook for Upper Back and Neck Pain (2nd ed., 2013) Anchorage: Institute of Trigger Point Studies (e-book, Print-on-Demand)

Trigger Point Therapy Workbook for Shoulder Pain including Frozen Shoulder (2nd ed., 2013) Anchorage: Institute of Trigger Point Studies (e-book, Print-on-Demand)

Trigger Point Therapy Workbook for Lower Back and Gluteal Pain (2nd ed., 2013) Anchorage: Institute of Trigger Point Studies (e-book, Print-on-Demand)

Trigger Point Therapy Workbook for Chest and Abdominal Pain (2013) Anchorage: Institute of Trigger Point Studies (e-book)

Trigger Point Therapy Workbook for Headaches & Migraines including TMJ Pain (2013) Anchorage: Institute of Trigger Point Studies (e-book, Print-on-Demand)

Trigger Point Therapy Workbook for Lower Arm Pain including Elbow, Wrist, Hand & Finger Pain (2013) Anchorage: Institute of Trigger Point Studies (e-book, Print-on-Demand)

Copyright © 2024 Valerie DeLaune, LAc

Trigger Point Therapy Workbook for Knee, Leg, Ankle, and Foot Pain (2018) Anchorage: Institute of Trigger Point Studies (e-book, Print-on-Demand)

For more information on how to purchase these books, and for additional resources, go to http://triggerpointrelief.com/

"Like" the *author* on Facebook at Facebook.com: Valerie-DeLaune

"Like" the *Institute of Trigger Point Studies* on Facebook at Facebook.com: Institute-of-Trigger-Point-Studies

www.ingramcontent.com/pod-product-compliance
Lightning Source LLC
Chambersburg PA
CBHW081201020426
42333CB00020B/2585